Low-FODMAP DIET COOKBOOK for Beginners

CATHERINE WADE

Table of Contents

Your Free Gift..1

Introduction... 3

Who Can Benefit from a Low-FODMAP Diet? 5

Benefits 7

Cultivating the Right Mindset Before Starting the FODMAP Diet 9

Understanding FODMAPs 11

What Are FODMAPs? 13

How Does the FODMAP Diet Work?.....................................17

Safe to Eat..19

Food Stacking Warning...21

Elimination Phase 22

Reintroduction Phase 25

Maintenance Phase... 29

Avoiding Confusion... 31

Meal Plans, Shopping Lists and Recipes............................. 35

WEEK 1...**37**

7-Days Meal Plan 38

Shopping List... 39

    Sunflower Seed Butter & Strawberry Sandwich....................40

    Toasted Walnuts 41

    Fruity Kiwi Smoothie 42

    Poached Eggs & Toast.. 43

    Spinach Scrambled Eggs with Orange & Papaya 44

    Macadamia Nuts 45

    Walnuts.. 45

    Strawberry Chia Coconut Dream 46

    Mushroom & Tofu Scramble 47

    Strawberry Papaya Smoothie....................................... 48

    Strawberry Lemon Pancakes 49

    Bagel & Scrambled Eggs 50

Buttery Shrimp with Boiled Potatoes...51

Mini Eggplant Pizzas...52

Tuna & Potato Salad...53

One Pan Salmon with Green Beans & Roasted Tomato...54

Brown Rice...55

Maple Mustard Chicken with Green Beans...56

Quinoa...57

Creamy Coconut Chicken with Rice...58

Ginger Salmon Patties with Fennel & Cucumber Salad...59

Poached Cod in Tomato Sauce with Spaghetti...60

Celery Root Latkes & Beef Patties...61

Meatballs & Carrot Mash...62

Baked Potato...63

Mediterranean Pasta with Kale...64

Grilled Eggplant with Spiced Walnuts & Yogurt...65

Baked Pizza Chicken...66

Potato Patties...67

Cheezy Broccoli Quinoa...68

Sweet & Spicy Candied Pecans...69

Cucumber Tuna Bites...70

Cucumber & Herbed Yogurt Dip...71

Cheese & Carrot Balls...72

Salted Peanut Fat Bombs...73

Vanilla Rice Pudding...74

Strawberry Lime Popsicles...75

WEEK 2...77

7-Days Meal Plan...78

Shopping List...79

Strawberry Buckwheat Pancakes...80

Tuna & Goat Cheese Egg Muffins...81

Pineapple Cucumber Smoothie...82

Tomato & Brie Omelet...83

Pineapple Lime Smoothie...84

Cinnamon Maple Brown Rice Porridge 85

Kale & Mozzarella Egg Muffins 86

Eggs in a Hole 87

Strawberry Orange Smoothie 88

Coconut Chia Seed Yogurt 89

Tofu Veggie Wrap 90

Air Fryer Lemon Dill Chicken Wings 91

Boiled Potato 92

Lemon & Cilantro Baked Pickerel 93

One Pot Cheeseburger Pasta 94

Steak, Mashed Potatoes & Green Beans 95

Coconut Cod & Spinach with Rice 96

Roasted Potato Frittata 97

Carrot Salad 98

Beef Meatballs 99

Mackerel Fish Cakes 100

Mashed Carrots 101

One Pan Roasted Tahini Chicken & Potato 102

Shrimp, Kale & Quinoa Salad 103

Coconut Yogurt Chicken 104

Crispy Eggplant Fries 105

Chicken & Quinoa Meatballs 106

Pan Fried Zucchini 107

Creamy Herb Chicken Lettuce Wraps 108

Macadamia Nut Clusters 109

Creamy Spiced Broccoli 110

Cheezy Walnuts 111

Pineapple Chia Pudding 112

Radish & Cucumber Rice Cakes 113

Sea Salted Coconut Kale Chips 114

Tropical Fruit Salad 115

WEEK 3 . . . . **117**

7-Days Meal Plan 118

Shopping List. 119

    Coconut Yogurt Parfait. 120

    Sweet & Savory French Toast 121

    Sheet Pan Strawberry Pancakes. 122

    Pineapple Yogurt Bowl. 123

    Pumpkin Seeds Spoons 124

    Air Fryer Broccoli & Cheddar Quiche Cups. 125

    Coconut Matcha Latte. 126

    Flourless Peanut Butter Pancakes. 127

    Golden Smoothie 128

    Plain Omelet with Cucumber 129

    Sweet & Sour Chicken with Broccoli. 130

    Carrot & Parsley Omelet. 131

    Chicken Fingers & Fries 132

    Strawberry Kiwi Salad with Chicken 133

    Greek Pasta Salad. 134

    Tofu Veggie Fried Rice 135

    Broccoli, Chicken & Cheese Melt. 136

    Walnut Crusted Salmon 137

    Mashed Potatoes. 138

    Maple Dijon Chicken & Lemon Herb Rice. 139

    Lemony Shrimp Pasta. 140

    Marinated Eggplant with Quinoa. 141

    Chicken & Potato Casserole 142

    Broiled Lemon & Pepper Sole 143

    Slow Roasted Salmon with Citrus 144

    Pineapple with Cinnamon 145

    Sea Salt Spinach Chips 146

    Radishes & Swiss Cheese 147

    Sesame Cucumber Salad. 148

    Dark Chocolate Peanut Butter Cups. 149

    Orange Popsicles. 150

Kiwi, Yogurt & Maple Syrup..151

WEEK 4 153

7-Days Meal Plan 154

Shopping List..155

Coconut Plantain Pancakes 156

Kiwi Green Smoothie....................................157

Warm Parsley Tomato Plantain Wrap 158

Coconut Matcha Smoothie........................... 159

Tuna Rice Cake.. 160

Maple Walnut Millet Porridge 161

Steak & Potato Egg Muffins 162

Turmeric Quinoa Breakfast Bowls 163

Orange Creamsicle Chia Pudding 164

Pumpkin Seeds Cup 165

Creamy Dill Salad with Chicken 166

Spinach Tuna Crepes.................................. 167

Broiled Mackerel 168

Curried Kale Salad.................................... 169

Cajun Chicken, Potatoes & Kale 170

Grilled Tempeh & Eggplant with Rice................. 171

Pan Fried Tofu Spinach Salad 172

Meatball Lettuce Wraps............................... 173

Massaged Kale Salad with Salmon 174

Potato Shepherd's Pie................................ 175

Baked Cilantro Lime Chicken......................... 176

Tomato & Thyme Quinoa 177

Maple Beef Burgers 178

Herbed Rice.. 179

Zucchini & Tuna Pasta Salad 180

Cumin Roasted Chicken & Broccoli................... 181

Pan-Fried Trout with Herbed Rice 182

Papaya with Yogurt & Walnuts 183

Frozen Coconut Yogurt Covered Strawberries 184

Kiwi & Strawberries. 185

Lemon Dill Yogurt Dip & Carrots. 186

Orange & Strawberry Frozen Yogurt Bites 187

Cucumbers & Salmon Dip. 188

Brazilian Cheese Bread. 189

BONUS RECIPES. 191

Chocolate & Strawberry Yogurt Bark 192

Lemon Coconut Power Balls 193

Dark Chocolate Peanut Mousse 194

Coconut Yoghurt Chia Pudding 195

Double Chocolate Mug Cake 196

Orange Cantaloupe Smoothie. 197

Strawberry & Peanut Butter Smoothie 198

Dragon Fruit & Kiwi Smoothie. 199

Zucchini Parmesan Muffins 200

Vanilla Mint Matcha Creamsicles 201

Balsamic Tomato & Basil Mini Egg White Bites. 202

Salmon Stuffed Cherry Tomatoes 203

Broccoli & Cheddar Egg Muffins. 204

Salmon Tartare & Tortilla Chips. 205

Cheeseburger Soup. 206

Food Translations. 207

Cooking Conversions 208

Your Free Gift

On your journey through the low-FODMAP Diet, diligent tracking of your diet and symptoms is paramount. As a thank you for purchasing my book, I've prepared printable resources for your convenience to assist you in this crucial endeavor.

To get instant access go to: https://cw.squarereads.com

The Food & Symptom Tracker printable download includes:

- Daily Tracker
- Monthly Symptom Tracker
- Safe / Suspect Food List
- Notes

You can organize these printable pages within a ring binder, and methodically document every aspect of your journey. This meticulous record-keeping will prove invaluable in your quest for digestive wellness.

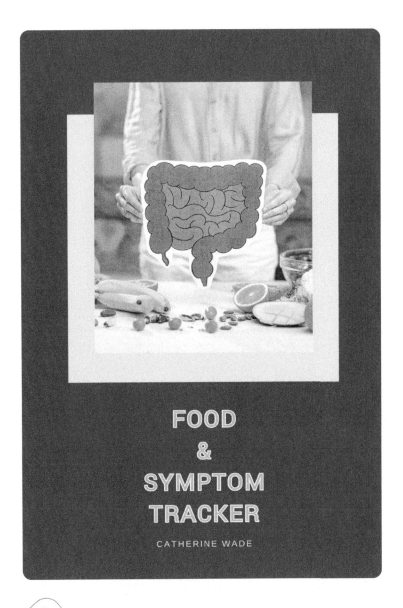

FOOD & SYMPTOM TRACKER

CATHERINE WADE

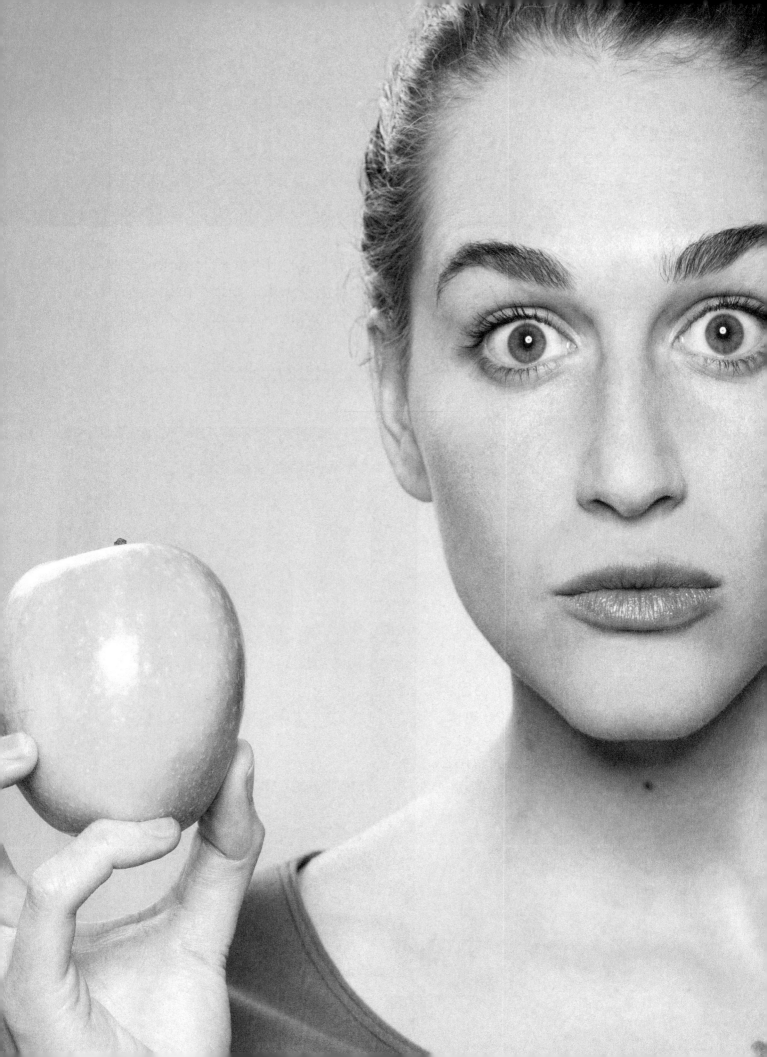

Introduction

We all know eating a healthy, balanced diet is good for us. After all, an apple a day keeps the doctor away.

But what if this isn't always the case?

We are all unique individuals, and the food we eat impacts our lives. As we are all unique, what is good for you isn't necessarily good for me, which can result in all sorts of issues.

So how do you know which food is causing you the problem?

The only way to know for sure is to use a process of elimination. It's like a detective eliminating a list of suspects. Everyone associated with the victim can be considered a suspect at first, but during the investigation, one by one, suspects are eliminated until the real culprit is found.

So, in the beginning, all foods are suspect. Until your investigation is complete, you won't know which one to eliminate, even foods considered healthy, like the apple.

That is where the FODMAP diet comes in.

In the book, you will see references to Monash University, the authority on the FODMAP diet.

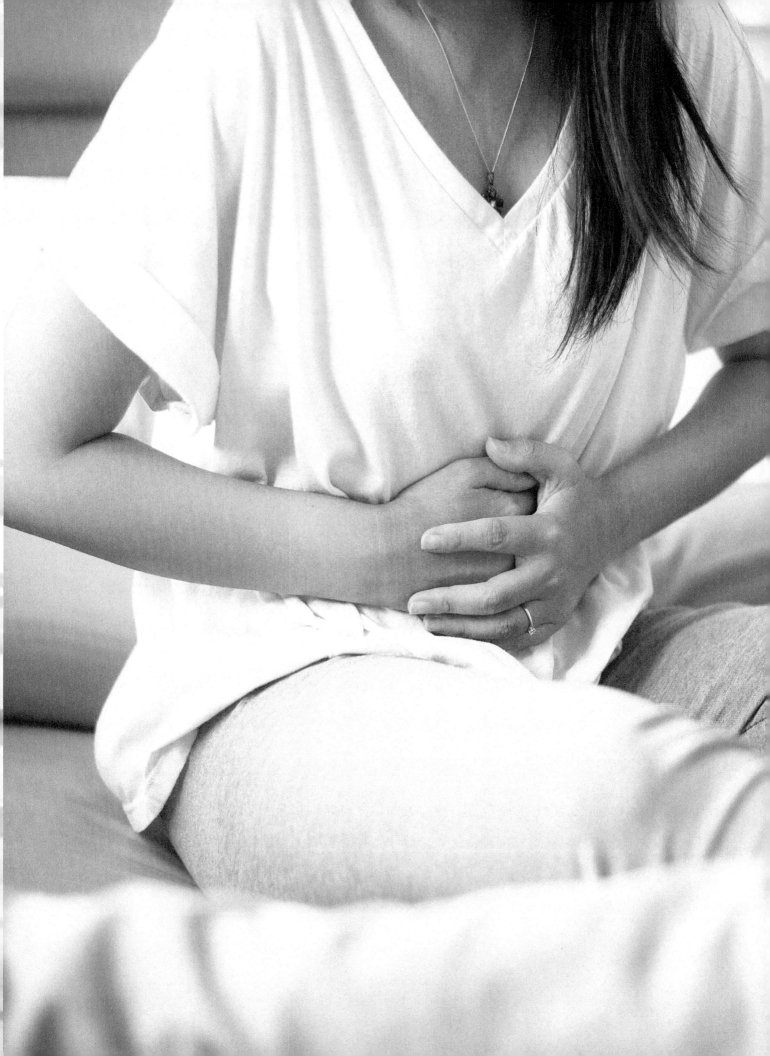

Who Can Benefit from a Low-FODMAP Diet?

The FODMAP diet is primarily recommended for individuals who experience recurring digestive symptoms like bloating, gas, abdominal pain, and altered bowel habits, particularly those diagnosed with IBS. However, working with a healthcare professional before starting the diet is recommended to ensure it suits your condition.

OTHER CONDITIONS THE FODMAP DIET CAN HELP

While the FODMAP diet was initially developed to alleviate symptoms in individuals with Irritable Bowel Syndrome (IBS), its benefits have also extended to other conditions.

Inflammatory Bowel Disease (IBD)

Some people with Crohn's disease or Ulcerative Colitis, both forms of Inflammatory Bowel Disease, may experience digestive symptoms similar to those seen in IBS. The FODMAP diet can assist in identifying trigger foods and providing relief from abdominal discomfort, bloating, and diarrhea, which are common symptoms of IBD.

Functional Gut Disorders

Apart from IBS, other functional gastrointestinal disorders share similar symptoms. Sufferers from conditions like Functional Dyspepsia, characterized by ongoing pain or discomfort in the upper abdomen, and small intestinal bacterial overgrowth (SIBO), where bacteria flourish in the small intestine causing bloating and diarrhea, might benefit from FODMAP dietary adjustments.

Non-Gastrointestinal Symptoms

Some individuals might experience non-gastrointestinal symptoms, like headaches or fatigue, that seem unrelated to the gut. However, evidence suggests a connection between the gut and other bodily systems. A FODMAP diet might be worth exploring to determine if certain foods contribute to these symptoms.

Athletes and Endurance Training

Athletes, particularly endurance athletes, often struggle with gastrointestinal issues during training and competitions. While the FODMAP diet may not be a solution for everyone, reducing high-FODMAP foods could minimize gut discomfort during intense physical activities.

Bloating and General Discomfort

Excessive bloating, gas, and general gut discomfort can be bothersome even for individuals without diagnosed digestive conditions. Exploring a low-FODMAP diet on a short-term basis may help identify foods that contribute to these symptoms and lead to a more comfortable everyday life.

Consulting a healthcare professional before making any dietary changes is crucial, as they can help determine whether the FODMAP diet is appropriate for your specific situation and guide you through the process to ensure balanced nutrition while managing symptoms.

Benefits

The FODMAP diet can offer a range of benefits for those struggling with digestive discomfort, particularly those suffering from IBS and other related conditions.

KEY BENEFITS

Reduced Digestive Symptoms

The FODMAP diet primarily aims to alleviate gastrointestinal symptoms such as bloating, gas, abdominal pain, and irregular bowel habits. By identifying and avoiding specific trigger foods, individuals often experience a significant reduction in these uncomfortable symptoms.

Personalized Approach

The FODMAP diet is not a one-size-fits-all solution. It's designed to be tailored to your specific sensitivities and tolerances. You can pinpoint the exact FODMAPs that trigger your symptoms through the Elimination and Reintroduction phases, creating a personalized dietary plan.

Improved Quality of Life

Chronic digestive discomfort can impact your daily life significantly. By managing your symptoms through the FODMAP diet, you can experience an improved overall quality of life, allowing you to engage in activities without being limited by digestive issues.

Better Nutritional Awareness

Following the FODMAP diet requires careful attention to ingredient labels and food choices. This heightened awareness often leads to a better understanding of nutritional content and the potential to make healthier food choices in the long run.

Less Dependency on Medications

For some individuals, the FODMAP diet can help reduce the need for medications to manage gastrointestinal symptoms. By addressing the root cause through diet, you might rely less on medications to control discomfort.

Potential Insights into Other Conditions

Beyond IBS, the FODMAP diet has shown promise in managing symptoms of other gastrointestinal disorders and even non-gastrointestinal conditions, such as migraines and fatigue, which might have an underlying gut connection.

Gastrointestinal Healing

Giving your gut a break from high-FODMAP foods during the Elimination Phase allows your digestive system to heal, contributing to a healthier gut environment over time.

Increased Energy

Many individuals report feeling more energetic and less tired after successfully identifying and eliminating FODMAP triggers from their diet. Reduced digestive distress can lead to improved overall energy levels.

Enhanced Body-Mind Connection

The FODMAP diet encourages mindfulness about how your body reacts to different foods. This heightened awareness can lead to a better understanding of the body-mind connection and the effect food has on your feelings.

Long-Term Management

By identifying and managing your specific FODMAP triggers, you will gain valuable knowledge to apply over the long-term, allowing you to enjoy a wider variety of foods while avoiding those that cause discomfort.

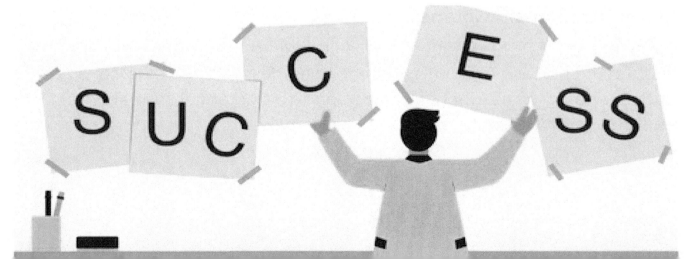

Cultivating the Right Mindset Before Starting the FODMAP Diet

Embarking on the FODMAP diet can be a transformative journey towards improved digestive health. However, success on this path often begins with the right mindset. Developing a positive and proactive attitude can make the process smoother and more effective.

Here's how to foster the right mindset before starting the FODMAP diet:

Educate Yourself

Knowledge is your ally to understand FODMAPs, why they might trigger your symptoms, and how the diet works. Empower yourself with accurate information to confidently approach the diet and clearly understand its purpose.

Be Patient

Rome wasn't built in a day, and digestive healing won't happen overnight, either. The FODMAP diet involves different phases, and each step has its role in uncovering triggers and building a personalized eating plan. Approach the journey patiently, knowing that long-term benefits often require gradual adjustments.

Stay Open-Minded

You'll be exploring new foods and rethinking your eating habits. Stay open to trying new ingredients and recipes. This isn't about depriving yourself. It's about discovering delicious and gut-friendly options you might not have considered before.

Embrace the Experiment

The FODMAP diet is, in essence, an experiment with your body. It's a journey of self-discovery. Not every food will affect you the same way as it does others.

So track your reactions, and keep a food diary, which can help you fine-tune your diet effectively.

Focus on What You Can Eat

Instead of fixating on what you're temporarily eliminating, switch your focus to the abundance of foods you can enjoy. Explore low-FODMAP options and discover a world of nutritious and delicious ingredients that are friendly to your digestive system.

Practice Self-Compassion

This journey isn't about perfection. There might be moments when you inadvertently consume high-FODMAP foods or experience setbacks. Instead of being harsh on yourself, practice self-compassion. Remember that setbacks are part of the learning process.

Stay Curious

The FODMAP diet is about more than just food. It's about understanding your body and its responses.

Stay curious about how different foods affect you. Use this knowledge to make informed choices that promote your well-being.

Celebrate Small Wins

Celebrate every milestone, whether completing the Elimination Phase or identifying trigger foods during reintroduction. These achievements are steps toward a healthier you.

Visualize Your Goal

Picture yourself enjoying improved digestive comfort and a better quality of life. Visualizing what you are trying to achieve can help you stay motivated, especially during challenging moments.

Approaching the FODMAP diet with the right mindset sets the stage for success. Remember, you're taking control of your health and well-being. By being patient, open-minded, and well-informed, you're laying the foundation for positive changes that can impact your digestive health and overall wellness.

Understanding FODMAPs

FODMAPs consist of fermentable short-chain carbohydrates. In simpler terms, this signifies two crucial characteristics: firstly, they are sugar molecules organized in chains, and secondly, they are susceptible to fermentation by the bacteria residing in your gut. When molecules are connected in chains, they require enzymatic breakdown into single molecules before they can be absorbed efflciently through your small intestine.

Several digestive challenges may arise when your body encounters difflculty breaking down these chain-like FODMAP molecules into their individual components. These undigested chains continue their journey into the large intestine, serving as a feast for the resident gut bacteria. As these bacteria feast on the FODMAPs, they produce gases as byproducts. This gaseous production can cause the intestines to expand and stretch, leading to sensations of abdominal bloating and distension.

In addition, undigested FODMAPs in the large intestine can draw water into the bowel, potentially causing diarrhea or altered bowel habits. Consequently, the inability to effectively break down these carbohydrates into single molecules can result in various gastrointestinal discomforts and symptoms. This is particularly relevant for individuals with conditions like Irritable Bowel Syndrome (IBS), where the FODMAP diet can provide relief by pinpointing specific trigger foods and alleviating these digestive issues.

When foods rich in FODMAPs enter the small intestine, they continue into the large intestine (colon), largely intact because these carbohydrates aren't well absorbed in the small intestine.

In the colon, FODMAPs become a feast for gut bacteria. As these bacteria ferment the undigested carbohydrates, they produce gas as a byproduct. This gas can cause the intestines to expand, leading to feelings of abdominal distension and bloating.

Additionally, FODMAPs have an osmotic effect, meaning they draw water into the intestines. This often results in diarrhea or loose stools for some individuals, while others may experience constipation.

The combination of gas production, water retention, and changes in bowel habits can lead to abdominal discomfort or pain. Over time, these symptoms can contribute to exhaustion and fatigue as the body copes with digestive distress.

It's important to remember that not everyone is equally sensitive to FODMAPs, and the severity of symptoms will vary from person to person. The FODMAP diet can offer relief for IBS sufferers by identifying and managing specific trigger foods to minimize these uncomfortable gastrointestinal symptoms.

In the following chapters, we'll delve deeper into each phase of the FODMAP diet, providing practical tips, recipes, and guidance to make your journey smoother.

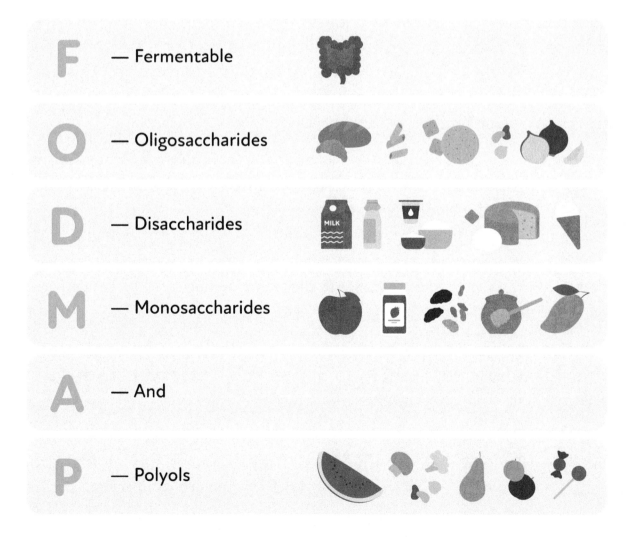

F — Fermentable

O — Oligosaccharides

D — Disaccharides

M — Monosaccharides

A — And

P — Polyols

What Are FODMAPs?

FODMAPs are carbohydrates that are not easily broken down by bacteria in the gut, leading to gas production, discomfort, and abdominal issues.

F: Fermentable

O: Oligosaccharides

D: Disaccharides

M: Monosaccharides

A: and

P: Polyols

Fermentable

The "F" in FODMAP stands for fermentable, which refers to the process by which gut bacteria break down undigested carbohydrates, producing gas and other byproducts. While all FODMAPs are fermentable, the specific types listed below can be problematic for people with sensitive guts.

Oligosaccharides

Oligosaccharides are short-chain carbohydrates made up of a few sugar molecules linked together. They include various types of carbohydrates, such as fructans and galacto-oligosaccharides (GOS). When poorly absorbed in the small intestine, gas and bloating are caused as they ferment in the large intestine. Some foods fall under both Fructans and GOS.

FRUCTANS

Artichokes	Cashews	Garlic
Asparagus	Cauliflower	Inulin Supplements
Bananas (ripe)	Cherries	Leeks
Blueberries	Chickpeas	Legumes
Broccoli (stalks)	Chicory Root	Lentils
Cabbage	Dates	Mushrooms

Nectarines	Pistachios	Scallions	Watermelon
Onions	Raspberries	Shallots	Wheat
Pears	Rye	Snow Peas	

GOS

Cashews

Cow's Milk: it's essential to differentiate between lactose (a disaccharide) and galactose (a component of GOS) when considering dairy products)

Legumes: lentils, chickpeas, and beans (black beans, kidney beans)

Legume-Based Products: hummus (made from chickpeas) and some veggie burgers (containing legume ingredients)

Pistachios

Snow Peas

Soy-Based Products: soybeans, soy milk, tofu

Disaccharides

Disaccharides include double sugar molecules such as lactose, commonly found in dairy products.

Lactose intolerant individuals experience diffculty digesting lactose, creating gas and diarrhea.

The three significant disaccharides are sucrose, lactose, and maltose.

Lactose is the primary disaccharide of concern in the FODMAP diet. Reintroducing disaccharides, specifically lactose, can help you identify whether you have lactose intolerance or sensitivity.

Foods Containing Disaccharides

Buttermilk	Dairy Milk (cow's, goat's)	Soft Cheeses (ricotta, cottage)
Condensed Milk	Evaporated Milk	
Cream Cheese	Ice Cream	Sour Cream
Cream	Processed Foods (dressings, ready mixes)	Yogurt

Monosaccharides

Fructose and glucose are monosaccharide sugars. These are single sugar molecules, like fructose, in fruits and honey.

FRUCTOSE

Fruits (apples, pears, cherries, mangoes, watermelons)
Fruit Juices (apple, pear)
Honey

High-Fructose Corn Syrup (HFCS), a sweetener used in processed foods and beverages
Agave Syrup (often used as a sweetener)
Broccoli (stalks), Broccolini (heads)

GLUCOSE

Glucose is a monosaccharide found naturally in various foods, mainly carbohydrates. These foods naturally contain glucose as a component of their carbohydrate content. Glucose, a primary energy source for our bodies, is readily absorbed into the bloodstream to provide energy to cells.

Bananas	Lychees	Honey
Grapes	Sweet Potatoes	Sport's Drinks
Cherries	Peas	Energy Gels
Dates	Oats	Dextrose (sweetener)
Raisins	White Bread	
Prunes	Pasta	

Polyols

Polyols, also known as sugar alcohols, naturally occur in some fruits and vegetables and are used as artificial sweeteners in sugar-free products. Polyols are sugar alcohols in some fruits and artificial sweeteners like sorbitol and xylitol. Common polyols include sorbitol (in apples, pears) and mannitol (in mushrooms, cauliflower).

Check ingredients on any food items you buy as you do not want to buy anything containing:

Xylitol

Xylitol is commonly found in sugar-free gum, candies, and dental products like toothpaste and mouthwash. It is also used as a sweetener in some sugar-free baking and cooking recipes.

Erythritol

Erythritol, a sugar alcohol, is often used as a sweetener in various sugar-free and low-calorie foods and beverages. It's often found in sugar-free gum, candies, and baking products.

Sorbitol

Sorbitol is found naturally in some fruits but is often used as a sugar substitute in sugar-free and reduced-sugar foods. It's frequently used in sugar-free chewing gum and sugar-free candies.

Mannitol

Mannitol is used as a sugar substitute in sugar-free and reduced-sugar products. It is also used in some medications and medical preparations.

Isomalt

Isomalt is regularly used as a sugar substitute in sugar-free candies and other confectionery products. It is often used to create sugar-free hard candies.

Lactitol

Lactitol is a sugar alcohol used in some sugar-free and reduced-sugar foods. It is used in sugar-free ice cream and dairy-based products.

Maltitol

Maltitol is a sugar alcohol commonly used in sugar-free and reduced-sugar candies, chocolates, and baked goods.

Hydrogenated Starch Hydrolysates (HSH)

HSH is a group of sugar alcohols used as sweeteners in various sugar-free and reduced-sugar food products.

Maltitol Syrup

This sweet syrup from maltitol is used in sugar-free and reduced-sugar food products, particularly syrups and toppings.

Polyols that remain unabsorbed within the small intestine proceed into the large intestine, where they undergo fermentation by the resident gut bacteria. This bacterial fermentation generates gas as a byproduct, leading to the distension of the bowel and resulting in added discomfort, bloating, and changes in bowel patterns for individuals prone to such effects.

Polyols can draw water into the intestines, potentially leading to diarrhea and gas in sensitive individuals.

Now that you understand what FODMAPs are, it's time to understand how the FODMAP diet actually works.

How Does the FODMAP Diet Work?

The FODMAP diet involves eliminating high-FODMAP foods for a specific period, usually 2 – 6 weeks, to help identify which FODMAPs might be causing your digestive discomfort.

The FODMAP diet consists of three phases:

1. Elimination Phase
2. Reintroduction Phase
3. Maintenance Phase

It's important to note that the FODMAP content of foods can vary, and portion sizes also play a role. Although some foods may be tolerated well in small amounts, they can trigger symptoms when consumed in larger quantities. The FODMAP diet involves a structured approach to identify individual tolerance levels.

It is vital to avoid FODMAP stacking, where you eat more than one food from a FODMAP group.

Remember, the goal of the FODMAP diet isn't to eliminate these carbohydrates forever but to determine which ones are causing discomfort and create a balanced eating plan that minimizes symptoms while still allowing for a variety of nutrient-rich and enjoyable foods in your diet.

Keep a Food Diary

Maintain a detailed food diary to track your meals, symptoms, and emerging patterns. This can help you and your dietitian fine-tune your diet during the Reintroduction Phase. This diary is invaluable for tracking your reactions to specific foods.

Seek Support

Share your dietary journey with friends and family so they can offer support and understanding. Joining FODMAP diet support groups or online communities can provide valuable advice and encouragement.

Seek Professional Guidance

It's important to note that while the FODMAP diet can offer significant benefits, it's not suitable for everyone, and individual responses vary. Consulting a healthcare professional before making any dietary changes is essential to ensure that the FODMAP diet is appropriate for your specific situation and health needs.

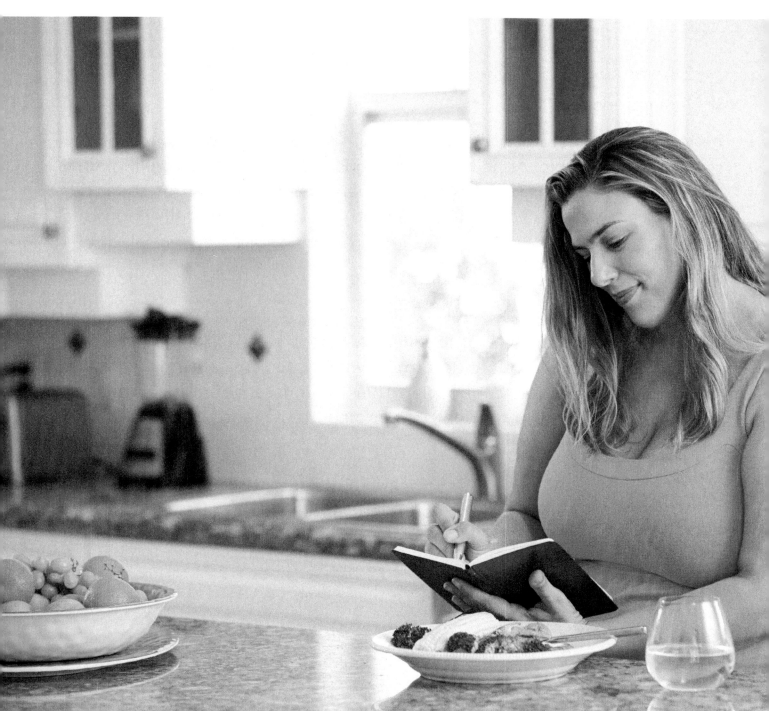

Safe to Eat

Effectively navigating the FODMAP diet involves knowing which foods are low in FODMAPs, allowing you to create a balanced and symptom-friendly meal plan. Below, you'll find an extensive list of low-FODMAP foods categorized into different groups, which will aid you in planning meals and snacks that align with your dietary requirements.

Remember, portion size is key.

Vegetables

Bell Peppers (red no FODMAPs, half a green is Low-FODMAP)
Carrots
Cucumbers
Eggplant
Green Beans (15 beans)
Lettuce
Spinach
Tomatoes
Zucchini
Potatoes (small)
Bok Choy
Chives
Ginger
Olives (small amount)
Pumpkin (less than half a cup)
Turnips
Bamboo Shoots
Chard
Choy Sum
Kale
Radishes
Seaweed (nori)
Spring Onions (green part)

Fruits

Blueberries (20 berries)
Grapes (1 cup)
Kiwi
Lemon
Lime
Oranges
Pineapple (1 cup)
Raspberries (1/3 cup)
Strawberries
Bananas (unripe)
Cantaloupe
Honeydew Melon
Passion Fruit
Rhubarb

Dairy

Lactose-free Milk
Hard Cheeses (cheddar,
    mozzarella, parmesan – 1/4 cup)
Lactose-free Yogurt
Butter

Protein

Chicken (skinless)
Eggs
Fish
Lamb
Pork (lean cuts)
Tofu (firm)
Turkey
Beef (lean cuts)
Seafood (crab, lobster, shrimp)

Grains and Cereals

Oats (limited serving)
Quinoa
Rice (white, brown, limited serving)
Polenta
Cornflour
Gluten-free Pasta
    (made from rice, corn, or quinoa)
Rice Cakes

Nuts and Seeds

Almonds (10 almonds)
Brazil Nuts
Macadamia Nuts
Pumpkin Seeds
Sunflower Seeds
Walnuts
Pine Nuts
Pecans

Beverages

Black Tea (limited)
Coffee (limited)
Green Tea
Herbal Teas (peppermint,
    chamomile)
Water
Almond Milk (unflavored, limited)
Coconut Water (limited)
Club Soda
Grape Juice (limited)
Orange Juice (limited small
    servings)
Pineapple Juice (limited)

Condiments and Flavor Enhancers

Maple Syrup (limited)
Olive Oil
Salt and Pepper
Spices (cinnamon, cumin, paprika,
    etc.)
Mayonnaise (moderate, with no
    garlic, onion)
Mustard
Soy Sauce (limited)
Vinegar (limited)
Miso Paste (limited)
Fish Sauce (limited)
Tomato Paste

Sweets and Snacks

Dark Chocolate (limited)
Popcorn (plain)
Rice Crackers
Potato Chips (plain, limited)
Rice Crisps

Food Stacking Warning

Food stacking, in the context of the FODMAP diet, refers to consuming multiple servings of similar low-FODMAP foods within a short time frame, which can result in the cumulative intake of FODMAPs that may trigger digestive symptoms.

- When you consume a meal or snack, it's essential to consider the FODMAP content of individual foods and their cumulative effect.

- Some low-FODMAP foods can become high in FODMAPs when consumed in large quantities or when multiple servings are eaten in quick succession.

- The key FODMAPs to watch out for in this context are fructans (found in wheat, garlic, onion, etc.), polyols (like sorbitol and mannitol found in certain fruits and vegetables), and fructose (found in some fruits).

Food stacking can lead to gastrointestinal discomfort, gas, bloating, and other symptoms, even if each food individually is considered low-FODMAP.

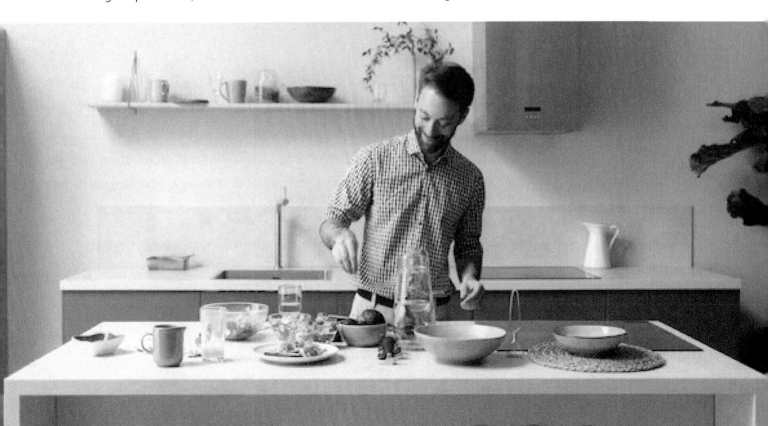

Elimination Phase

The Elimination Phase is the most challenging phase of the FODMAP diet. All your cooking habits, food choices, and go-to dishes are no longer an option. Although this can be a daunting phase, it can also be fun!

Think of all the new foods you might discover and how beneficial it will be to eliminate those problem foods and finally reduce your symptoms.

Follow the Elimination Phase for 2 - 6 weeks. During this phase, avoid high-FODMAP foods to give your gut a chance to calm down. You'll stick to a low-FODMAP diet, which means avoiding foods in the different FODMAP groups, including certain fruits, vegetables, dairy products, wheat, and some sweeteners.

As the name of this phase suggests, the goal here is to eliminate FODMAPS from your diet by only eating low-FODMAP or foods that are FODMAP-free. Fish and seafood are proteins and don't contain carbohydrates. As FODMAPs consist only of carbohydrates, protein foods are free from FODMAPs and can be eaten safely.

Make the process more manageable by following the 28-day Meal Plan outlined in this book, where a selection of balanced, delicious, and nutritious meals has been designed to ease you through this phase. Every ingredient in these recipes is compatible with the Elimination Phase. If you decide to continue beyond the initial 28 days, you can simply loop back to day one to maintain your progress.

At any time, if your symptoms have significantly improved, you can move on to the Reintroduction Phase.

If there is no improvement in your symptoms after six weeks, more than likely, FODMAPs are not the cause of your problem, and you should visit your health practitioner to discuss the matter further.

Use the following tips during the Elimination Phase.

Familiarize Yourself with High-FODMAP Foods

Learn which foods are high in FODMAPs and read food labels carefully. Common high-FODMAP foods include garlic, onions, wheat, certain fruits, and some dairy products.

Plan Your Meals in Advance

Create a meal plan or use the Meal Plan in this book for the Elimination Phase that includes low-FODMAP foods. By planning, you will find it easier to stick to your diet to ensure you always have suitable options available.

Batch Cooking

Cook in batches and freeze portions of low-FODMAP meals. This can save you time and effort on busy days and help prevent the temptation of high-FODMAP convenience foods.

Stock Your Pantry

Keep your pantry stocked with low-FODMAP staples like rice, gluten-free pasta, canned tomatoes, and canned tuna. Having these items on hand can simplify meal preparation.

Experiment with New Recipes

Embrace the opportunity to explore new recipes and cooking techniques. Many delicious dishes can be created using low-FODMAP ingredients.

Monitor Portion Sizes

While some high-FODMAP foods may be tolerated in small amounts, paying attention to portion sizes is crucial. Eating large quantities of even low-FODMAP foods can sometimes trigger symptoms.

Be Patient and Persistent

Digestive symptoms may not disappear immediately. Give your body time to adjust to the Elimination Phase. Keep going, even if it takes a little while to notice improvements.

Read Ingredient Labels

Check ingredient labels on packaged foods for hidden sources of high-FODMAP ingredients. Some processed foods may contain FODMAPs or additives that can trigger symptoms.

Stay Hydrated

Drink plenty of water throughout the day to help maintain digestive regularity and overall well-being.

Remember that the Elimination Phase is crucial in identifying trigger foods and finding relief from digestive symptoms. By following these tips and working closely with a healthcare professional, you can navigate this phase effectively and set the stage for a successful Reintroduction Phase.

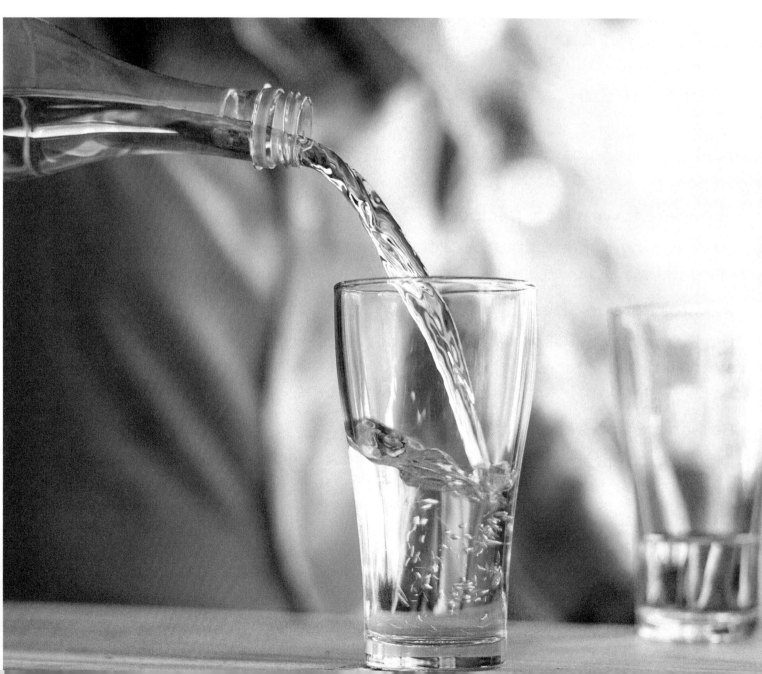

Reintroduction Phase

Once you have successfully completed a few weeks of the Elimination Phase, you'll move on to the Reintroduction Phase of the diet. In this phase, you reintroduce foods from one FODMAP group at a time, in controlled amounts, to identify which specific FODMAPs trigger your symptoms. This helps customize the diet to your tolerances.

To make this easier, refer to the chapter called *What Are FODMAPs?* You will find foods listed under each group to start eating again. You can still use the recipes provided but add your chosen ingredient. If your symptoms subsided during the Elimination Phase following the Meal Plan, and you experience no new symptoms when one item is reintroduced, this is probably a good indicator that you can safely eat that ingredient.

Here are some tips to help you navigate this phase effectively:

Reintroduce One FODMAP Group at a Time

Reintroduce ingredients from one FODMAP group at a time, starting with those you miss the most or suspect are less likely to trigger your symptoms. You'll eat one food from that group over three days, each day increasing the amount of the food you reintroduce. Over time, introduce more and more ingredients from the different food groups. Food lists can be found in the chapter *What Are FODMAPs?* Please refer to the chapter *Avoiding Confusion* for insight regarding foods that fall into multiple FODMAP groups.

OLIGOSACCHARIDES

Start by reintroducing one group of oligosaccharides at a time. The main groups to consider are fructans and galacto-oligosaccharides (GOS).

When deciding which oligosaccharide group to begin with, your choice can be influenced by your personal preferences and dietary habits. For instance, if you often miss eating sandwiches, you should begin with fructans to assess your tolerance to wheat-based bread. Alternatively, if you want to add legumes to your meals, you might prioritize GOS.

Fructans are a group of oligosaccharides found in various foods, including wheat, onions, garlic, and certain fruits and vegetables. If you prioritize fructans, you might begin by reintroducing a small amount of wheat-based bread. This could involve consuming a single slice of wheat bread with your meal.

GOS are another group of oligosaccharides found in foods like legumes (lentils, chickpeas, beans), certain nuts, and vegetables like snow peas.

To reintroduce GOS, you might start with a small portion of cooked lentils. Begin with half a cup of cooked lentils added to a salad or soup.

DISACCHARIDES

Select one lactose-containing food from the food list. It's recommended to start with a small portion of a food you miss or believe is the least likely to trigger symptoms. If you experience symptoms, return to your baseline low-FODMAP diet until the symptoms resolve. Once you're symptom-free, you can proceed to the next reintroduction.

MONOSACCHARIDES

Understand which specific monosaccharides you want to reintroduce. The main monosaccharides are glucose and fructose. Choose either glucose or fructose to reintroduce first. It's best to focus on one at a time to pinpoint potential reactions. Pick a whole, unprocessed food source rich in the chosen monosaccharide. For glucose, options include dates, raisins, prunes, or sweet potatoes. For fructose, fruits like apples or watermelon are good choices. Start with a small portion of the chosen food source.

POLYOLS

Typical polyols include xylitol, erythritol, sorbitol, mannitol, isomalt, and lactitol. Choose one polyol to reintroduce initially. Focusing on one at a time helps identify any specific sensitivities. Choose a food or product that contains the selected polyol. For example, if you're reintroducing xylitol, you might start with sugar-free gum or candies sweetened with xylitol, or if you're reintroducing sorbitol, try sugar-free candies containing sorbitol.

REINTRODUCTION GUIDELINES

Monitoring and Progress

After reintroducing a food from your chosen group, carefully track your symptoms in a food diary. Note any digestive discomfort, such as bloating, gas, abdominal pain, or changes in bowel movements. Document the type and severity of symptoms and the timing of their onset. This information will be valuable in assessing your tolerance to specific foods.

Follow a Structured Plan

You can also work with a registered dietitian to create a structured reintroduction plan tailored to your needs and sensitivities. This plan should outline the order of reintroductions and the amounts to consume.

Gradually Increase Portion Sizes

Start with a small portion of the reintroduced food and gradually increase the amount over several days. This helps you pinpoint your tolerance level and the threshold at which symptoms occur.

Be Patient and Observant

Pay close attention to your body's response to each reintroduced food. Digestive symptoms may not appear immediately, so be patient and allow time for any delayed reactions to become apparent.

Use Pure Sources

When reintroducing a FODMAP group for the first time, choose foods that are a pure source of that group. For example, if reintroducing fructans, use a slice of wheat bread rather than a complex meal with multiple ingredients.

Don't Skip Reintroductions

It's essential to reintroduce all FODMAP groups, even if you believe you have no issues with certain types. This thorough process helps you identify specific trigger foods accurately.

Reintroduce Small Amounts of High-FODMAP Foods

For high-FODMAP foods you miss and wish to incorporate back into your diet, try reintroducing them in small amounts. You may find that you can tolerate limited quantities without triggering symptoms.

Reevaluate and Adjust

If a particular food or FODMAP group triggers symptoms, remove it from your diet again and wait until your symptoms subside. Returning to a three-day restriction phase between food reintroductions is recommended.

Be Mindful of Stress and Lifestyle Factors

Stress and lifestyle factors can impact digestive symptoms. Pay attention to how stress, sleep, and physical activity affect your reactions to reintroduced foods.

Remember that the Reintroduction Phase is the crucial part of the FODMAP diet. It helps you identify your dietary triggers and reintroduce a wider variety of foods while managing your digestive symptoms effectively.

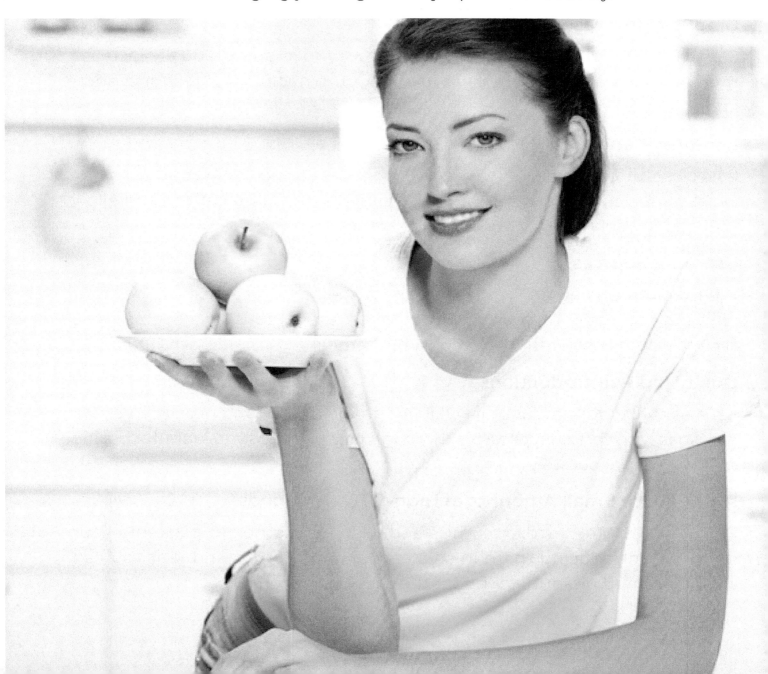

Maintenance Phase

Armed with knowledge about your FODMAP triggers, you can now create a long-term eating plan that minimizes your intake of high-FODMAP foods while allowing you to enjoy a wide variety of low-FODMAP options.

Congratulations!

You've completed the challenging but highly rewarding Elimination and Reintroduction Phases of the FODMAP diet. By now, you've likely identified your trigger foods and gained valuable insights into your digestive system.

Now, it's time to transition into the Maintenance Phase, where you'll focus on maintaining your newfound symptom relief and balanced nutrition.

Establish Your Personalized Diet

You've likely developed a tailored eating plan that suits your specific needs. Continue to follow this plan, emphasizing well-tolerated foods and avoiding your identified high-FODMAP trigger foods.

Keep a Food Diary

Maintaining a food diary can be beneficial even in the Maintenance Phase. It helps you track your diet, symptoms, and potential triggers that may have been missed during the Reintroduction Phase. This ongoing record can provide valuable insights and help you stay on track.

Monitor Portion Sizes

Be mindful of portion sizes, especially for foods that may still be high in FODMAPs but are well-tolerated in smaller quantities. Overindulging in these foods can lead to symptoms resurfacing.

Stay Informed

Keep yourself updated on the latest research and developments related to the low-FODMAP diet. While the core principles remain the same, new information may emerge that could enhance your management of digestive symptoms.

Seek Support and Professional Guidance

If you ever experience changes in your symptoms or have questions about your diet, don't hesitate to consult with your doctor or a dietitian. They can provide ongoing support, answer your questions, and adjust your diet plan.

Balance Nutrition

Maintaining a balanced diet is vital for your overall health. Ensure that you're getting a variety of nutrients from different food groups. Focus on foods low in FODMAPs and also rich in dietary fiber, vitamins, and minerals.

Enjoy the Benefits

The FODMAP diet isn't just about symptom relief but about improving the quality of your life. Use the knowledge you've gained to enjoy a wide range of foods without discomfort. Explore new recipes and cooking techniques that align with your dietary needs.

Stay Mindful

Digestive health is an ongoing journey. Practice mindfulness around eating, chew food thoroughly, and eat at a relaxed pace. These habits can contribute to improved digestion.

Remember that the Maintenance Phase is about finding a sustainable, long-term approach to managing your digestive symptoms. By staying informed, maintaining a balanced diet, and seeking professional guidance when needed, you can enjoy the benefits of the FODMAP diet and lead a more comfortable and fulfilling life.

Avoiding Confusion

There are a few foods that can cause confusion. You may believe they are high-FODMAP and, therefore, unsuitable for a low-FODMAP diet, but this is only sometimes the case. Some foods are low-FODMAP but, in larger quantities, are unsuitable to eat. Other foods may have a higher FODMAP count, but in very small amounts, they are suitable during the Elimination Phase.

BROCCOLI

Broccoli is a viable addition to your low-FODMAP meals, even during the Elimination Phase. It's worth noting that the florets and stems of broccoli have distinct FODMAP content, with the florets having lower levels. Consequently, the florets are a suitable choice for your low-FODMAP diet.

BANANAS

An unripe banana, weighing about 100 grams, has low levels of oligofructans, which makes it a safe choice for consumption on a low-FODMAP diet. However, it's important to note that a ripe banana contains high amounts of oligofructans, categorizing it as high in FODMAPs and, therefore, unsuitable for this diet.

BELL PEPPERS

According to Monash University, a low-FODMAP serving of red bell pepper is thought to be ⅓ cup or 43 grams. Green peppers are higher in FODMAPS, so be aware of portion sizes (about half is good). Yellow bell peppers have recently been tested again by Monash University. They are now considered low-FODMAP if the serving size is 24 grams.

WHITE BREAD

Monash has tested standard white bread (made of wheat) and is low in FODMAPs for one slice (24g). Even though it contains wheat, it has been processed and does not contain enough fructans to cause symptoms for most people with IBS.

MUSHROOMS

Oyster mushrooms are low-FODMAP in the amount specified in the Meal Plan. Other mushrooms are high-FODMAP.

GREEN BEANS

Green beans are low-FODMAP at 15 beans (75g) but contain moderate amounts of FODMAPs at 25 beans (125g), so make sure you watch your portion size.

BUTTER

Butter is low-FODMAP in typical serving sizes. Butter is primarily fat, and is very low in lactose, making it low-FODMAP.

MULTIPLE FODMAP GROUPS

As previously mentioned in the Reintroduction Phase chapter, some foods contain FODMAPs from more than one group, along with the specific FODMAP groups they belong to:

Wheat-Based Products (Fructans and Fructose)

Wheat contains fructans (an oligosaccharide) and fructose (a monosaccharide), placing wheat-based products, such as bread and pasta, in both the oligosaccharide and monosaccharide FODMAP groups.

Onions and Garlic (Fructans and Fructose)

Onions and garlic are known for their high content of both fructans (oligosaccharides) and fructose (monosaccharides), classifying them as high-FODMAP foods in both the oligosaccharide and monosaccharide categories.

Honey (Fructose and Fructans)

Honey contains elevated levels of both fructose (a monosaccharide) and excess fructose in the form of fructans (oligosaccharides), making it a high-FODMAP food in both the monosaccharide and oligosaccharide FODMAP groups.

Mangoes (Fructose and Sorbitol)

Mangoes contain fructose (a monosaccharide) and sorbitol (a polyol), categorizing them as high-FODMAP foods in both the monosaccharide and polyol FODMAP groups.

Watermelons (Fructose and Sorbitol)

Like mangoes, watermelons contain fructose (a monosaccharide) and sorbitol (a polyol), placing them in the monosaccharide and polyol FODMAP groups.

Cherries (Fructose and Sorbitol)

Cherries are another example of fruits containing both fructose (monosaccharide) and sorbitol (polyol), making them high-FODMAP foods in both the monosaccharide and polyol FODMAP groups.

Cashews (Excess Fructose and Mannitol)

Cashews contain excess fructose (in the form of fructans, an oligosaccharide) and mannitol (a polyol), categorizing them in both the oligosaccharide and polyol FODMAP groups.

These foods pose additional challenges for individuals following the FODMAP diet as they contain FODMAPs from multiple categories, increasing the likelihood of triggering digestive symptoms. During the Reintroduction Phase, it's advisable to test these foods individually to determine which specific FODMAPs within them are problematic for you and in what quantities. Consulting with a registered dietitian can provide expert guidance for managing your diet effectively.

Having explained all that, let's get into the nutritious low-FODMAP Meal Plans.

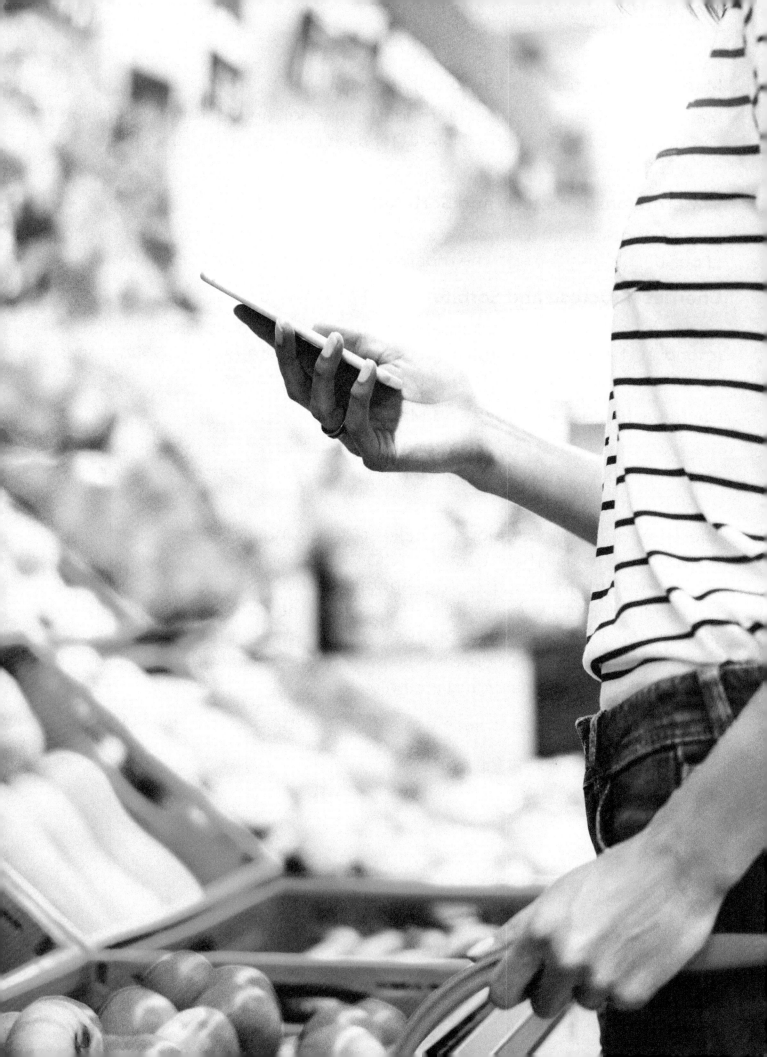

Meal Plans, Shopping Lists and Recipes

These are general meal plans not customized for your specific needs. They don't consider personal health issues, conditions, goals, other food intolerances, or allergies. This balanced and nutritious low-FODMAP Meal Plan should be used in the Elimination Phase.

The following 28-Day Meal Plan is divided into three four weekly sections.

1. 7-Days Meal Plan
2. Shopping List
3. Recipes

Each week includes daily breakfast, lunch, dinner, and snack recipes. The snack can be eaten anytime. All the food for each day has been nutritionally balanced, and this information is displayed. We all have days where we sometimes require more food, and with this in mind, you can have something from the *Bonus Recipes* or *Safe to Eat* chapters. When deciding what to have from these chapters, please do not choose anything containing the same ingredients in your Meal Plan for the day to avoid food stacking.

When you first start your Meal Plan, there will be ingredients on your shopping list that you probably do not already have in your pantry. However, many of these won't have to be repurchased as they will become part of your pantry staples as only a little will be used.

Do not be alarmed if any of the foods listed in the chapter *What Are FODMAPS?* are included in the Meal Plan. As frequently mentioned throughout this book, the quantity eaten determines whether it is safe on a low-FODMAP diet.

All the recipes in the specified quantities are low-FODMAP.

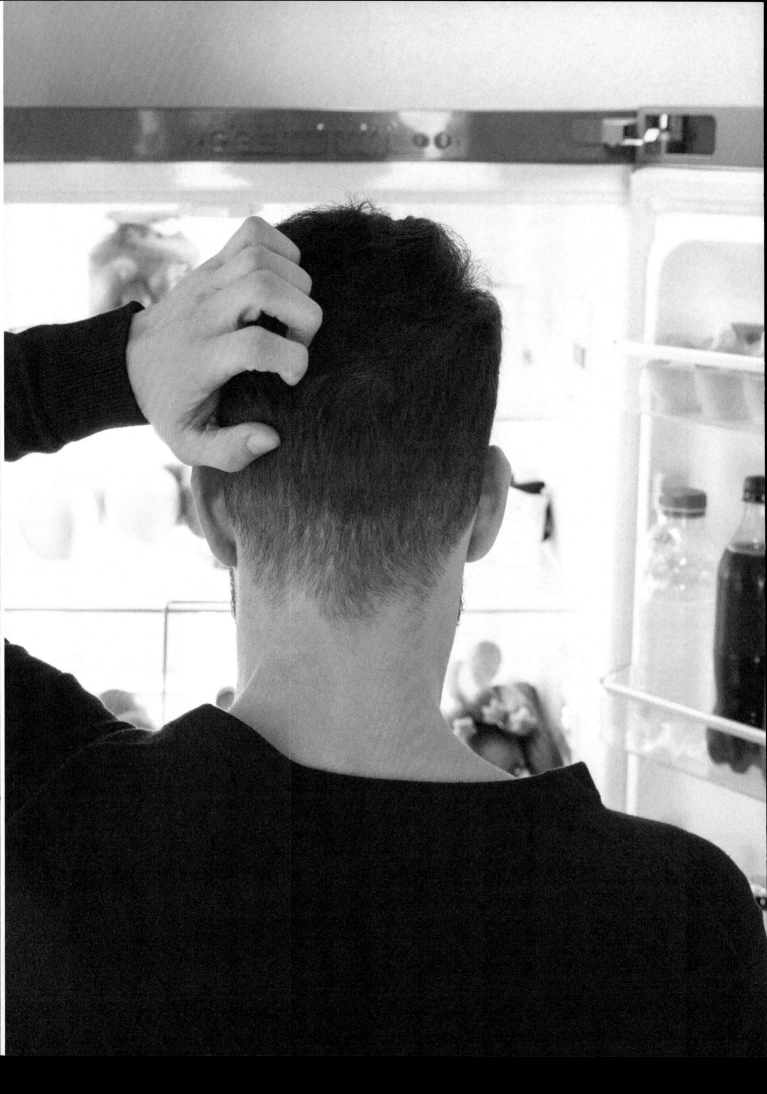

WEEK 1

Every recipe states the total number of servings and the total prep time so that you know how many servings the recipe creates, and how long it will take you to make it.

Before you start cooking, assemble all ingredients and prep them according to the ingredients list.

You will be eating one serving of each meal, even if the recipe serves more than one.

7-Days Meal Plan

MONDAY

BREAKFAST
Sunflower Seed Butter & Strawberry Sandwich, Toasted Walnuts

LUNCH
Buttery Shrimp with Boiled Potatoes

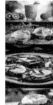

DINNER
Poached Cod in Tomato Sauce with Spaghetti

SNACKS
Sweet & Spicy Candied Pecans

TUESDAY

BREAKFAST
Fruity Kiwi Smoothie, Poached Eggs & Toast

LUNCH
Mini Eggplant Pizzas

DINNER
Celery Root Latkes & Beef Patties

SNACKS
Cucumber Tuna Bites

WEDNESDAY

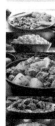

BREAKFAST
Spinach Scrambled Eggs with Orange & Papaya, Macadamia Nuts

LUNCH
Tuna & Potato Salad

DINNER
Meatballs & Carrot Mash, Baked Potato

SNACKS
Cucumber & Herbed Yogurt Dip

THURSDAY

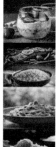

BREAKFAST
Strawberry Chia Coconut Dream

LUNCH
One Pan Salmon with Green Beans & Roasted Tomato, Brown Rice

DINNER
Mediterranean Pasta with Kale

SNACKS
Cheese & Carrot Balls

FRIDAY

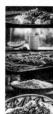

BREAKFAST
Mushroom & Tofu Scramble, Strawberry Papaya Smoothie

LUNCH
Maple Mustard Chicken with Green Beans, Quinoa

DINNER
Grilled Eggplant with Spiced Walnuts & Yogurt

SNACKS
Salted Peanut Fat Bombs

SATURDAY

BREAKFAST
Strawberry Lemon Pancakes

LUNCH
Creamy Coconut Chicken with Rice

DINNER
Baked Pizza Chicken, Potato Patties

SNACKS
Vanilla Rice Pudding

SUNDAY

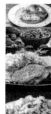

BREAKFAST
Bagel & Scrambled Eggs, Walnuts

LUNCH
Ginger Salmon Patties with Fennel & Cucumber Salad

DINNER
Cheezy Broccoli Quinoa

SNACKS
Strawberry Lime Popsicles

Shopping List

FRUITS
1 Kiwi
1 ¼ Lemon
2 1/3 tbsps Lemon Juice
1 ⅓ Lime
1 ½ tsps Lime Juice
½ Navel Orange
1 ½ cups Papaya
1 cup Pineapple
400 grams Strawberries

SEEDS, NUTS & SPICES
1/16 tsp Cayenne Pepper
2 ⅓ tbsps Chia Seeds
1/16 tsp Cinnamon
¾ tsp Cumin
⅛ tsp Dried Dill
½ tsp Italian Seasoning
⅓ cup Macadamia Nuts
¼ tsp Oregano
¼ cup Pecans
¼ tsp Red Pepper Flakes
Sea Salt & Black Pepper
¼ tsp Turmeric
120 grams Walnuts

FROZEN
9 Ice Cubes

VEGETABLES
3 cups Baby Spinach
1 tbsp Basil Leaves
75 grams Broccoli
6 Carrots
1 cup Celery Root
1 cup Cherry Tomatoes
1 tbsp Cilantro
1 ½ Cucumbers
150 grams Eggplant
½ bulb Fennel
⅓ cup Fresh Dill

1 ½ tsps Ginger
150 grams Green Beans
3 cups Kale Leaves
2 cups Mini Potatoes
2 tbsps Mint Leaves
¾ cup Oyster Mushrooms
3 ¼ tbsps Parsley
1 ½ Russet Potatoes
1 Yellow Potato

PANTRY STAPLES
2 ⅔ tbsps Arborio Rice
½ cup Brown Rice
113 grams Brown Rice Fettuccine
¼ cup Brown Rice Spaghetti
½ cup Canned Coconut Milk
¼ cup Jasmine Rice
1 ¼ cups Quinoa
1 ½ cans Tuna
¼ cup Vegetable Broth
¼ cup All Natural Peanut Butter
¼ cup Maple Syrup

BAKING
1 ⅓ tsps Baking Powder
⅔ cup Brown Rice Flour
2 ¾ tbsps Nutritional Yeast
1/16 tsp Stevia Powder
2 tbsps Unsweetened Shredded Coconut
1 ⅔ tsps Vanilla Extract

BREAD, FISH, MEAT & CHEESE
113 grams Cheddar Cheese
500 grams Chicken Breast
1 Cod Fillet
1 tbsp Cream Cheese, Regular
213 grams Extra Lean Ground Beef

114 grams Gluten-free Bagel
6 slices Gluten-free Bread
113 grams Lean Ground Beef
60 grams Mozzarella Ball
28 grams Mozzarella Cheese
370 grams Salmon Fillet
227 grams Shrimp
340 grams Tofu

CONDIMENTS & OILS
2 ¼ tbsps Apple Cider Vinegar
1 tbsp Avocado Oil
1 tbsp Capers
1 ½ tsps Coconut Aminos
2 ⅔ tbsps Coconut Oil
1 ½ tsps Dijon Mustard
½ cup Extra Virgin Olive Oil
¼ cup Pitted Kalamata Olives
1 ½ tsps Rice Vinegar
2 tbsps Sunflower Seed Butter
1 tbsp Tamari
1 ¼ cups Tomato Sauce

FRIDGE
2 ¾ tbsps Butter
14 Eggs
½ cup Orange Juice
1 cup Plain Coconut Milk
2 ½ cups Unsweetened Almond Milk
1 ⅛ cups Unsweetened Coconut Yogurt

Breakfasts

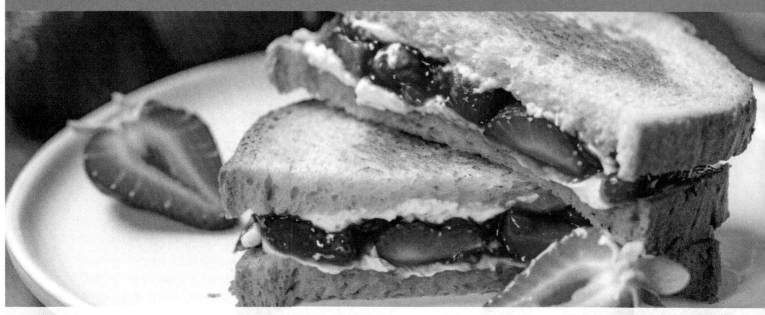

Sunflower Seed Butter & Strawberry Sandwich

 5 Minutes

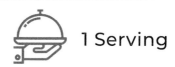 1 Serving

INGREDIENTS

- 2 slices Gluten-free Bread
- 2 tbsps Sunflower Seed Butter
- 1/4 cup Strawberries (stems removed, sliced)

INSTRUCTIONS

1. Toast the bread (optional).
2. Spread the sunflower seed butter onto the bread and top with sliced strawberries.
3. Close the sandwich and slice.

NUTRITION - AMOUNT PER SERVING

Calories	363	Sugar	10g
Fat	22g	Protein	9g
Carbs	35g	Cholesterol	0mg
Fiber	5g	Sodium	256mg

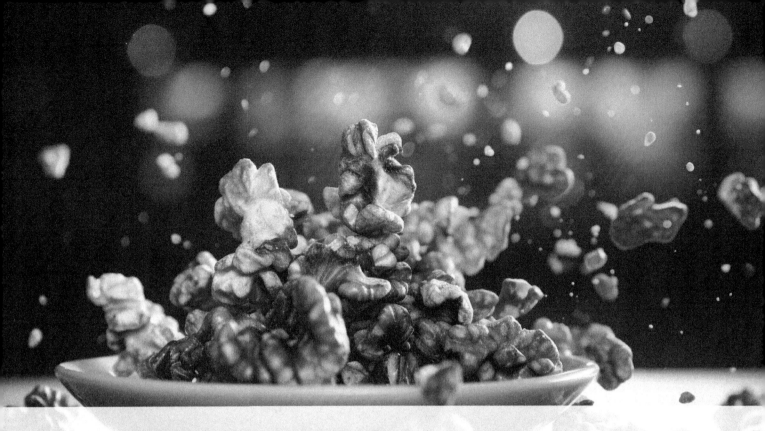

Toasted Walnuts

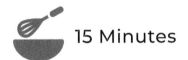 15 Minutes   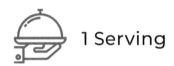 1 Serving

INGREDIENTS

- ⅓ cup Walnuts (shelled)

INSTRUCTIONS

1. Preheat oven to 350°F (177°C) and spread the walnuts across a baking sheet lined with parchment paper.

2. Toast in the oven for 5 to 10 minutes, tossing at the halfway point. Remove from oven, let cool and enjoy!

NUTRITION - AMOUNT PER SERVING

Calories	235	Sugar	1g
Fat	23g	Protein	5g
Carbs	5g	Cholesterol	0mg
Fiber	2g	Sodium	1mg

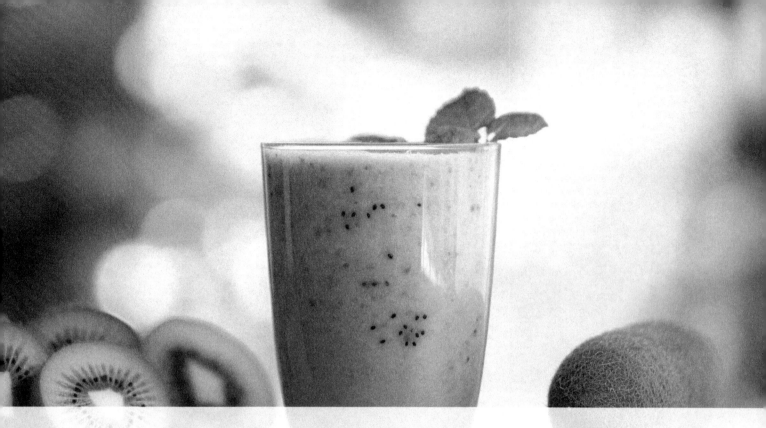

Fruity Kiwi Smoothie

 5 Minutes

 2 Servings

INGREDIENTS

- 1 Kiwi
- 1 cup Pineapple (fresh or frozen)
- 1 cup Kale Leaves
- ½ cup Unsweetened Coconut Yogurt
- ½ cup Orange Juice
- ½ cup Water
- 4 Ice Cubes

INSTRUCTIONS

1. Add all ingredients to a blender and blend until smooth.
2. Pour into a glass and enjoy!

NUTRITION - AMOUNT PER SERVING

Calories	121	Sugar	17g
Fat	2g	Protein	2g
Carbs	26g	Cholesterol	0mg
Fiber	3g	Sodium	22mg

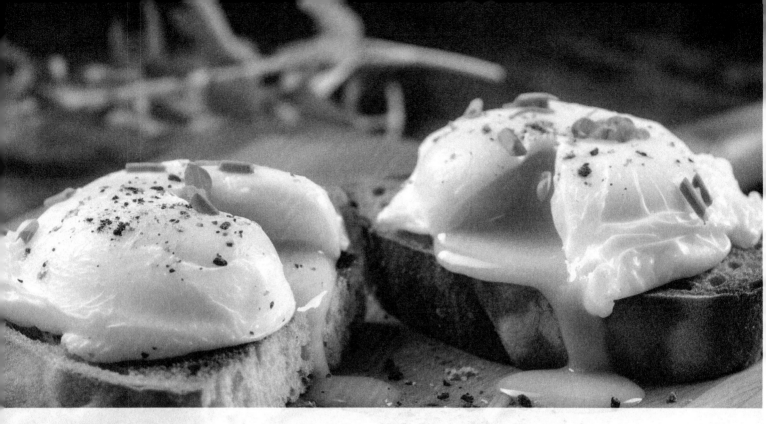

Poached Eggs & Toast

 10 Minutes

 2 Servings

INGREDIENTS

- 4 Eggs
- 2 tbsps Apple Cider Vinegar
- 4 slices Gluten-free Bread
- Sea Salt & Black Pepper

INSTRUCTIONS

1. Start by bringing a pot of water to a vigorous boil and incorporating the vinegar. Give the water a gentle stir with a spoon to generate a whirlpool effect.

2. Delicately place your eggs into the swirling water. Cook the eggs for about 3 to 4 minutes until they reach your preferred level of doneness.

3. Use a slotted spoon to retrieve the eggs from the water, and then let them rest on a plate lined with some paper towel before serving to absorb any excess moisture.

NUTRITION - AMOUNT PER SERVING

Calories	301	Sugar	5g
Fat	14g	Protein	16g
Carbs	25g	Cholesterol	372mg
Fiber	2g	Sodium	398mg

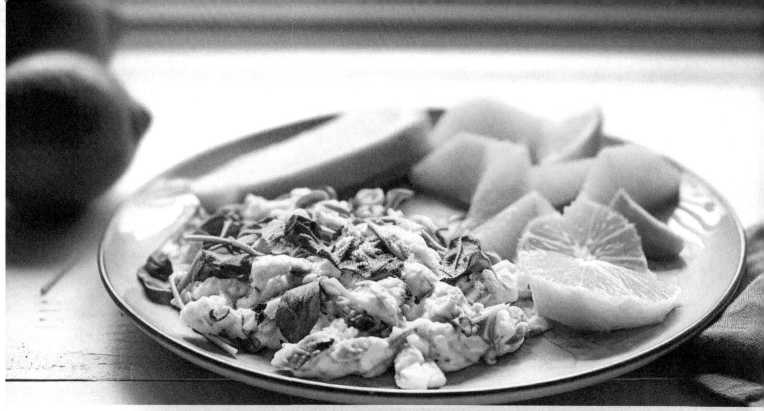

Spinach Scrambled Eggs with Orange & Papaya

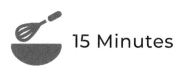 15 Minutes

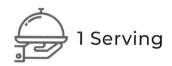 1 Serving

INGREDIENTS

- 2 Eggs
- 1 cup Baby Spinach (roughly chopped)
- 1 tbsp Fresh Dill (finely chopped)
- Sea Salt & Black Pepper (to taste)
- 1 tsp Butter
- ½ cup Papaya
- ½ Navel Orange (peeled and sectioned)

INSTRUCTIONS

1. Crack the eggs into a bowl and whisk well. Add the spinach, dill, salt, and pepper. Mix to combine.

2. Heat the butter in a pan over medium heat. Pour the egg mixture into the pan and scramble until it is cooked to your liking.

3. Add the scramble to a plate along with the papaya and orange.

NUTRITION - AMOUNT PER SERVING

Calories	248	Sugar	12g
Fat	14g	Protein	14g
Carbs	18g	Cholesterol	382mg
Fiber	3g	Sodium	173mg

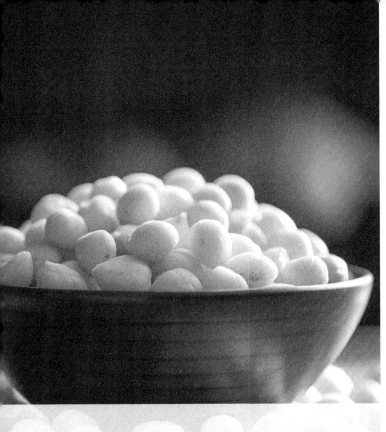

Walnuts

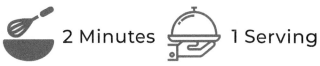

2 Minutes   **1 Serving**

INGREDIENTS   INSTRUCTIONS

- 30 grams
  Walnuts

1. Place in a bowl
   and enjoy!

NUTRITION - AMOUNT PER SERVING

Calories	196
Fat	20g
Carbs	4g
Fiber	2g
Sugar	1g
Protein	5g
Cholesterol	0mg
Sodium	1mg

Macadamia Nuts

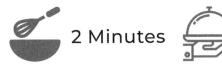

2 Minutes   **1 Serving**

INGREDIENTS   INSTRUCTIONS

- ⅓ cup
  Macadamia
  Nuts

1. Place in a bowl and
   enjoy!

NUTRITION - AMOUNT PER SERVING

Calories	321
Fat	34g
Carbs	6g
Fiber	4g
Sugar	2g
Protein	4g
Cholesterol	0mg
Sodium	2mg

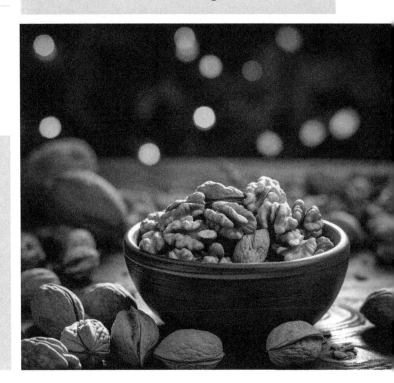

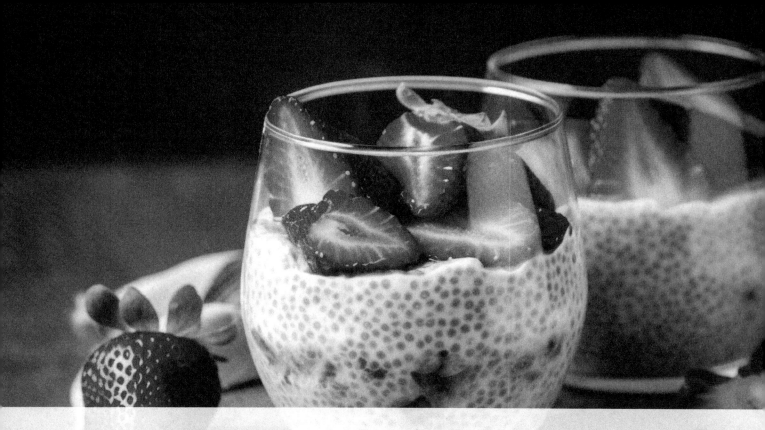

Strawberry Chia Coconut Dream

 35 Minutes

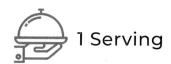 1 Serving

INGREDIENTS

- 1 cup Plain Coconut Milk
- 55 grams Strawberries (2 plus extra for garnish)
- 1 tsp Vanilla Extract
- 2 tbsps Chia Seeds
- 2 tbsps Unsweetened Shredded Coconut

INSTRUCTIONS

1. Add the coconut milk, strawberries, and vanilla to a small blender or food processor and blend well until combined.

2. Add the strawberry mixture to a medium-sized bowl and add the chia seeds. Stir well to combine. Refrigerate for at least 30 minutes or overnight to thicken.

3. Place the mixture in a bowl or in a to-go container. Top with extra strawberries (if using) and shredded coconut.

NUTRITION - AMOUNT PER SERVING

Calories	289	Sugar	11g
Fat	19g	Protein	5g
Carbs	24g	Cholesterol	0mg
Fiber	10g	Sodium	44mg

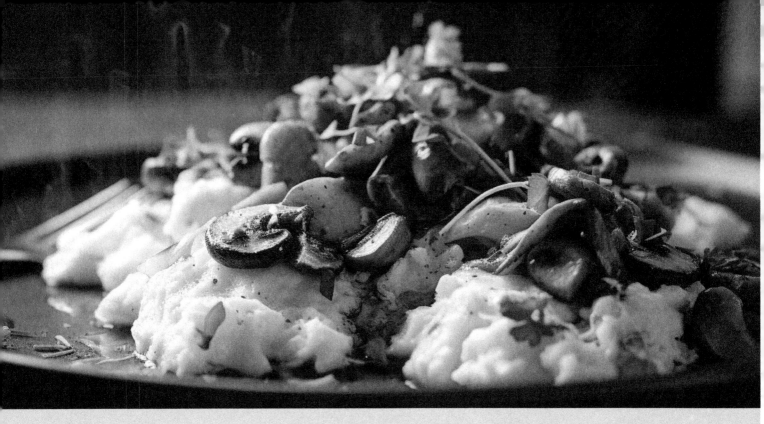

Mushroom & Tofu Scramble

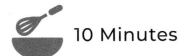 10 Minutes

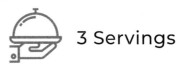 3 Servings

INGREDIENTS

- ¾ cup Oyster Mushrooms (sliced)
- ¼ cup Vegetable Broth (divided)
- 340 grams Tofu (extra firm, drained, crumbled)
- 1 tbsp Nutritional Yeast
- ¼ tsp Turmeric
- ¼ tsp Sea Salt

INSTRUCTIONS

1. Warm up a large skillet on medium heat for approximately 2 minutes. When it's ready, introduce the mushrooms and sauté them for 3 to 5 minutes, ensuring you stir them from time to time. If the mushrooms begin to stick, you can add half of the broth. Once done, transfer the mushrooms to a plate.

2. Now, in that same skillet, add the remaining portion of the broth, crumbled tofu, nutritional yeast, turmeric, and a pinch of salt. Stir the mixture and let it cook until the tofu is thoroughly heated.

3. Reintroduce the sautéed mushrooms to the skillet and blend them with the seasoned tofu. If you're on the move, portion the dish onto plates or into containers.

NUTRITION - AMOUNT PER SERVING

Calories	114	Sugar	1g
Fat	6g	Protein	14g
Carbs	4g	Cholesterol	0mg
Fiber	2g	Sodium	268g

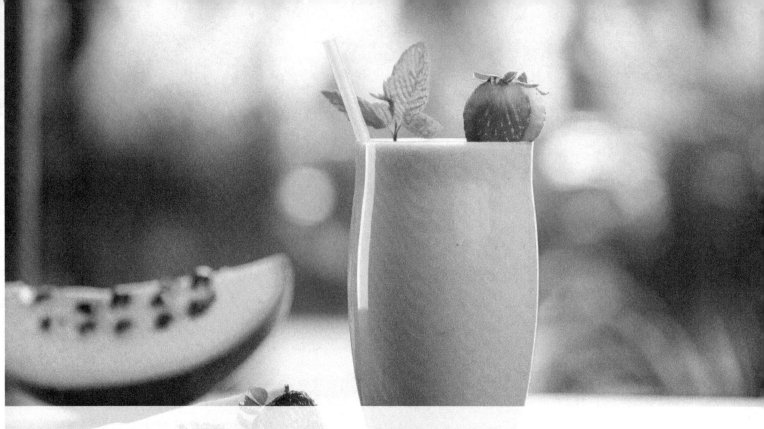

Strawberry Papaya Smoothie

 5 Minutes

 1 Serving

INGREDIENTS

- 1 cup Papaya
- ½ cup Strawberries (stems removed)
- ½ Lime (juiced)
- 1 cup Unsweetened Almond Milk
- 5 Ice Cubes

INSTRUCTIONS

1. Add all of the ingredients into a blender and blend until smooth.
2. Pour into a glass and enjoy!

NUTRITION - AMOUNT PER SERVING

Calories	118	Sugar	15g
Fat	3g	Protein	2g
Carbs	24g	Cholesterol	0mg
Fiber	5g	Sodium	137g

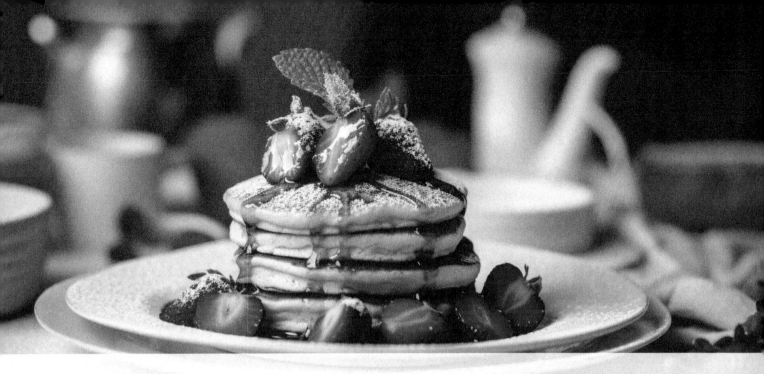

Strawberry Lemon Pancakes

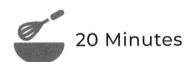 20 Minutes

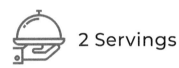 2 Servings

INGREDIENTS

- 2 Eggs
- ½ cup Unsweetened Almond Milk
- 1 ⅓ tbsps Maple Syrup
- 1 ⅓ tbsps Lemon Juice
- ⅔ cup Brown Rice Flour
- 1 ⅓ tsps Baking Powder
- 1/16 tsp Sea Salt
- 55 grams Strawberries (stems removed, chopped)
- 2 tsps Coconut Oil

INSTRUCTIONS

1. Whisk the eggs in a bowl. Incorporate the milk, maple syrup, and lemon juice, and stir well.

2. Introduce the flour, baking powder, and a pinch of salt into the mixture. Stir until you achieve a well-blended batter. Gently fold in the succulent strawberries.

3. Heat a pan over medium-high heat, adding a touch of oil. Scoop up about ¼ cup of batter at a time and pour it into the pan. Allow it to cook until you see bubbles emerging. Then, taking care, flip the pancakes and cook for an additional 1 to 2 minutes. Repeat this process with the remaining batter.

4. Divide the pancakes onto plates and enjoy every bite!

NUTRITION - AMOUNT PER SERVING

Calories	310	Sugar	10g
Fat	8g	Protein	6g
Carbs	53g	Cholesterol	62mg
Fiber	3g	Sodium	469mg

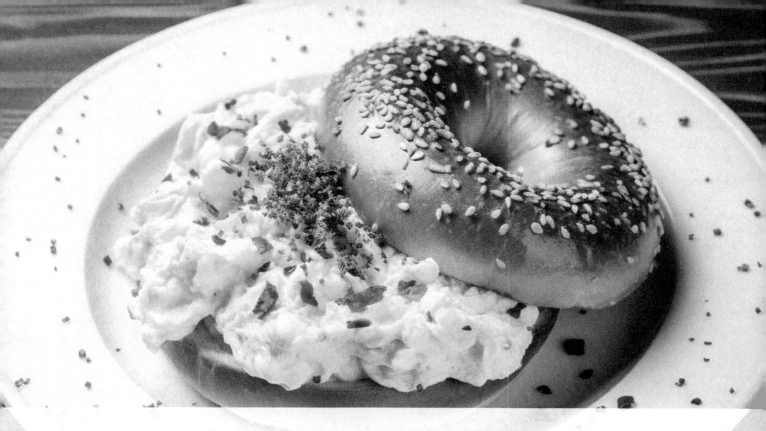

Bagel & Scrambled Eggs

 5 Minutes

 2 Servings

INGREDIENTS

- 114 grams Gluten-free Bagel (toasted)
- 1 tsp Extra Virgin Olive Oil
- 4 Eggs (whisked)
- Sea Salt & Black Pepper (to taste)

INSTRUCTIONS

1. Heat a pan over medium heat and add the oil. Add the whisked eggs to the pan and stir the eggs frequently as they cook.

2. Season with salt and pepper to taste.

3. To serve, place the egg and bagel on a plate and enjoy!

NUTRITION - AMOUNT PER SERVING

Calories	336	Sugar	7g
Fat	15g	Protein	15g
Carbs	34g	Cholesterol	374mg
Fiber	0g	Sodium	488mg

REFER TO PAGE 45 FOR THE ACCOMPANYING WALNUT RECIPE

Lunches

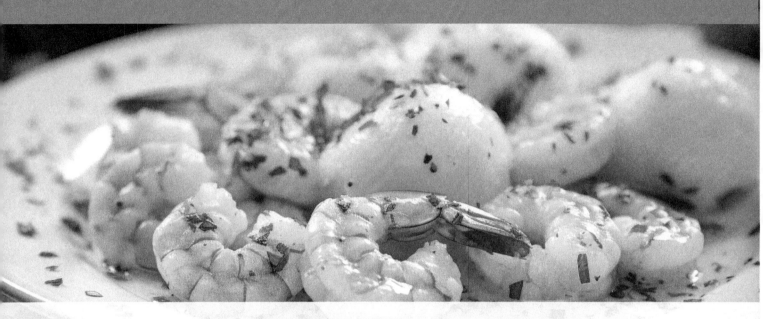

Buttery Shrimp with Boiled Potatoes

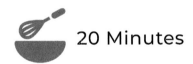 **20 Minutes**

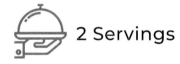 **2 Servings**

INGREDIENTS

- 1 Yellow Potato (medium, chopped)
- 2 tbsps Butter
- 227 grams Shrimp (peeled, deveined)
- 1/8 tsp Sea Salt

INSTRUCTIONS

1. Bring a large pot of water to a boil. Add the potatoes to the pot and boil for 15 minutes or until soft. Drain the water and set aside.

2. Meanwhile, melt the butter in a skillet over medium heat. Add the shrimp and cook for 1 to 3 minutes per side or until the shrimp are no longer translucent. Season with salt.

3. Divide the shrimp and potatoes onto plates.

NUTRITION - AMOUNT PER SERVING

Calories	280	Sugar	1g
Fat	12g	Protein	25g
Carbs	19g	Cholesterol	213mg
Fiber	2g	Sodium	290mg

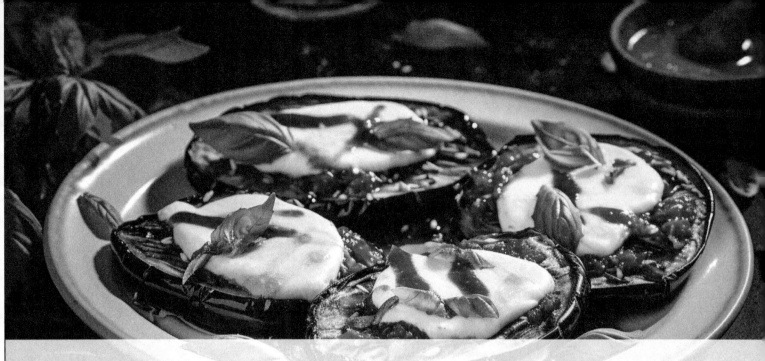

Mini Eggplant Pizzas

 30 Minutes

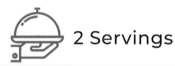 2 Servings

INGREDIENTS

- 75 grams Eggplant (medium)
- 2 tbsps Extra Virgin Olive Oil
- Sea Salt & Black Pepper (to taste)
- 1/3 cup Tomato Sauce
- 1/4 tsp Oregano
- 60 grams Mozzarella Ball (grated)
- 1/4 tsp Red Pepper Flakes (optional)
- 1 tbsp Basil Leaves (finely chopped)

INSTRUCTIONS

1. Begin by slicing the eggplant into uniform pieces, each about ½ inch thick. Coat both sides of the eggplant with a generous brushing of oil, and then season with sea salt and black pepper.
2. Warm a spacious non-stick pan over medium heat. Cook the eggplant slices in batches until they become tender which usually takes 3 to 5 minutes per side.
3. In the meantime, set your broiler to high.
4. Arrange the browned eggplant slices on a baking sheet, and generously layer each with tomato sauce, a sprinkle of oregano, and a blanket of shredded cheese. Slide the eggplant "pizzas" under the broiler for 3 to 5 minutes or until the cheese transforms into a gooey, bubbly, and enticing golden-brown topping.
5. To serve, finish with a pinch of red pepper flakes and a scattering of fresh basil.

NUTRITION - AMOUNT PER SERVING

Calories	230	Sugar	3g
Fat	20g	Protein	8g
Carbs	5g	Cholesterol	24mg
Fiber	2g	Sodium	151mg

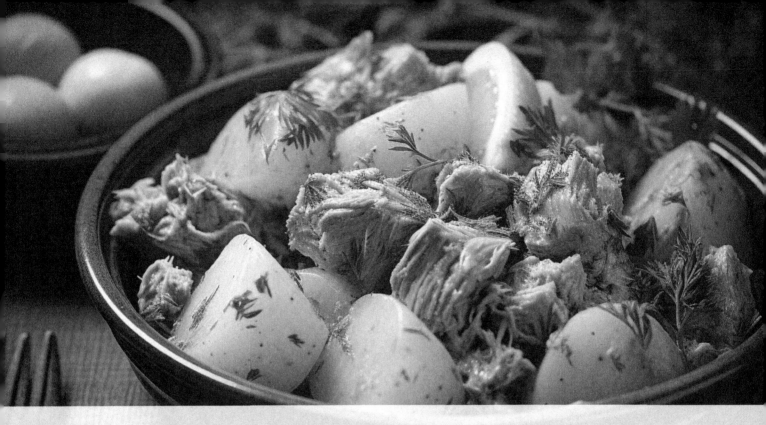

Tuna & Potato Salad

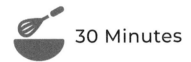 30 Minutes

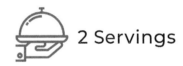 2 Servings

INGREDIENTS

- 2 cups Mini Potatoes
- 1 tbsp Capers (drained)
- 2 tbsps Extra Virgin Olive Oil
- 1 Lemon (medium, juiced)
- 2 tbsps Parsley (chopped)
- Sea Salt & Black Pepper (to taste)
- 1 can Tuna (drained)

INSTRUCTIONS

1. In a pot, add the potatoes making sure they are covered in water, and bring to a boil to cook for 12 to 15 minutes or until tender. Drain and let them cool before cutting them in half.

2. Place the cooked potatoes in a bowl and add the capers, oil, lemon juice, parsley, salt, and pepper. Flake the tuna and add it to the other ingredients in the bowl. Toss to combine.

3. Adjust the seasoning to your taste and enjoy!

NUTRITION - AMOUNT PER SERVING

Calories	313	Sugar	2g
Fat	15g	Protein	19g
Carbs	28g	Cholesterol	30mg
Fiber	4g	Sodium	316mg

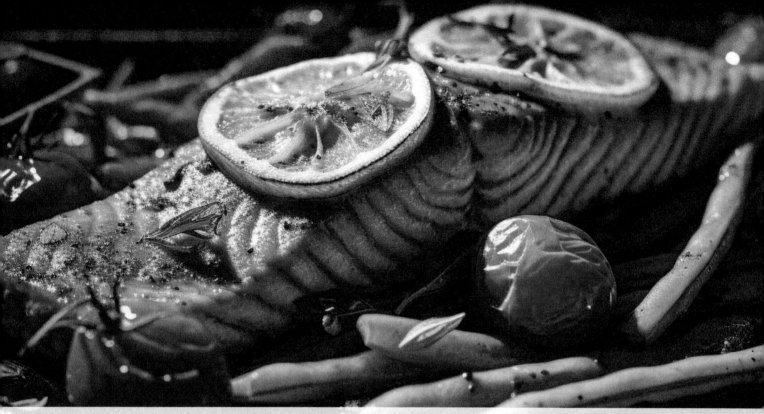

One Pan Salmon with Green Beans & Roasted Tomato

 25 Minutes

 2 Servings

INGREDIENTS

- 75 grams Green Beans (washed and trimmed)
- 1 cup Cherry Tomatoes
- 1 1/2 tsps Extra Virgin Olive Oil (or coconut oil)
- Sea Salt & Black Pepper (to taste)
- 200 grams Salmon Fillet

INSTRUCTIONS

1. Preheat oven to 428°F (220°C). Add the cherry tomatoes and green beans to a bowl, season with salt and pepper to taste, and toss with olive oil. Then, place on a baking sheet and bake for about 10 minutes.
2. Season your salmon fillets with sea salt and black pepper. Remove veggies from the oven and place salmon fillets over top. Return the dish to the oven and bake for a further 7 to 10 minutes or until the salmon flakes with a fork.
3. Divide veggies between plates and top with salmon.

NUTRITION - AMOUNT PER SERVING

Calories	186	Sugar	3g
Fat	8g	Protein	24g
Carbs	6g	Cholesterol	51mg
Fiber	2g	Sodium	84mg

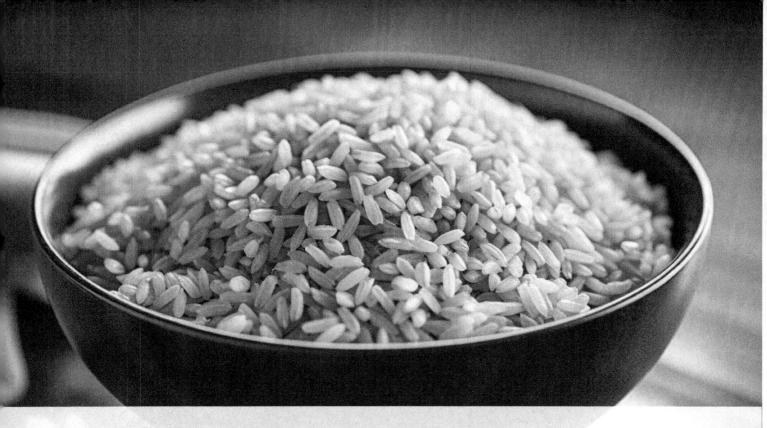

Brown Rice

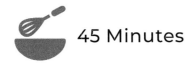 45 Minutes

 2 Servings

INGREDIENTS

- ½ cup Brown Rice (uncooked)
- 1 cup Water

INSTRUCTIONS

1. Combine the brown rice and water together in a saucepan. Place over high heat and bring to a boil.
2. Once boiling, reduce heat to a simmer and cover with a lid. Let simmer for 40 minutes or until water is absorbed.
3. Remove lid and fluff with a fork.

NUTRITION - AMOUNT PER SERVING

Calories	170	Sugar	0g
Fat	1g	Protein	3g
Carbs	35g	Cholesterol	0mg
Fiber	2g	Sodium	5mg

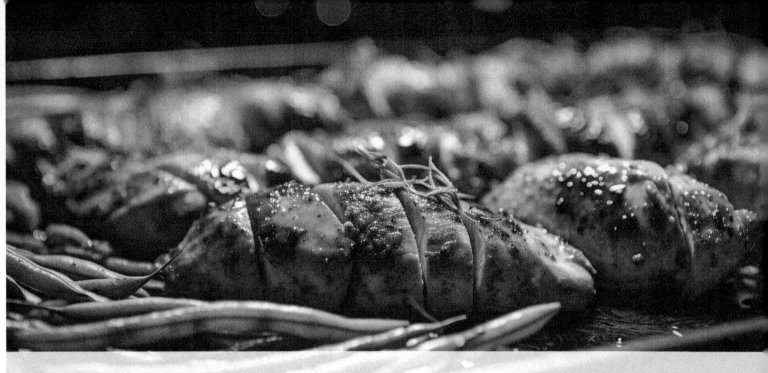

Maple Mustard Chicken with Green Beans

 25 Minutes

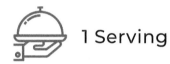 1 Serving

INGREDIENTS

- 1 1/2 tsps Maple Syrup
- 1 1/2 tsps Dijon Mustard
- 3/4 tsp Apple Cider Vinegar
- 1 1/2 tsps Tamari
- 160 grams Chicken Breast
- 75 grams Green Beans (washed and trimmed)
- 3/4 tsp Extra Virgin Olive Oil
- Sea Salt & Black Pepper (to taste)

INSTRUCTIONS

1. Mix a tangy marinade in a small bowl by combining maple syrup, dijon mustard, apple cider vinegar, and tamari. Whisk it well, then toss it into a ziplock bag with the chicken breasts. Give it a good shake and store it in the fridge.

2. Coat the green beans in extra virgin olive oil before seasoning with salt and pepper. Set them aside.

3. Fire up the grill to medium heat. Grill the chicken breasts for about 10 minutes per side until cooked through. Add the green beans to a grilling basket at the halfway mark and grill them for around 10 minutes, occasionally tossing.

4. Take the chicken and beans off the grill and serve them on plates.

NUTRITION - AMOUNT PER SERVING

Calories	285	Sugar	9g
Fat	8g	Protein	38g
Carbs	12g	Cholesterol	117mg
Fiber	2g	Sodium	663mg

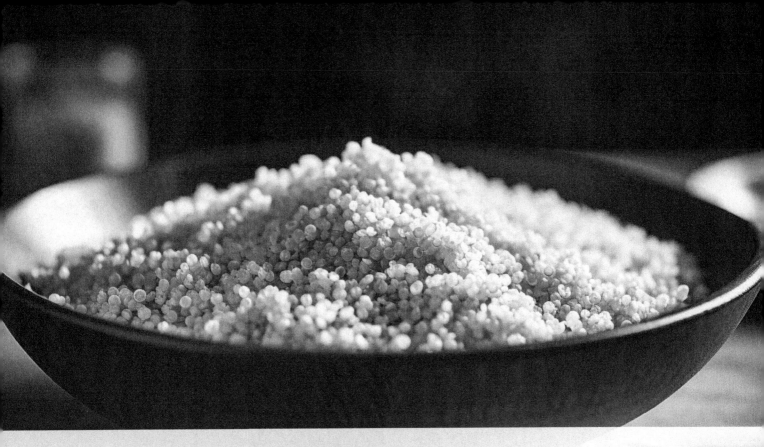

Quinoa

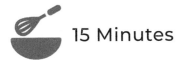 15 Minutes

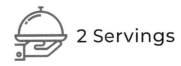 2 Servings

INGREDIENTS

- 1/2 cup Quinoa (uncooked)
- 3/4 cup Water

INSTRUCTIONS

1. Combine quinoa and water together in a saucepan. Place over high heat and bring to a boil. Once boiling, reduce heat to a simmer and cover with a lid.

2. Let simmer for 13 to 15 minutes or until water is absorbed. Remove lid and fluff with a fork.

NUTRITION - AMOUNT PER SERVING

Calories	156	Sugar	0g
Fat	3g	Protein	6g
Carbs	27g	Cholesterol	0mg
Fiber	3g	Sodium	4mg

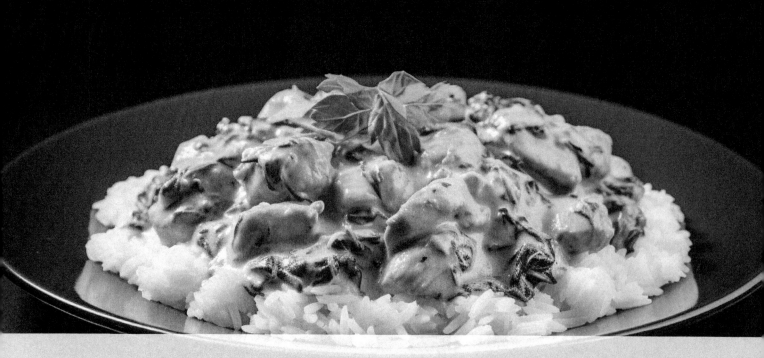

Creamy Coconut Chicken with Rice

 25 Minutes

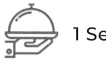 1 Serving

INGREDIENTS

- 1/4 cup Jasmine Rice (dry)
- 1/2 cup Canned Coconut Milk
- 1/4 cup Water
- 1 1/2 tsps Tamari
- 1 1/2 tsps Rice Vinegar
- Sea Salt & Black Pepper (to taste)
- 113 grams Chicken Breast (skinless, boneless, cubed)
- 2 cups Baby Spinach (chopped)

INSTRUCTIONS

1. Cook rice according to package instructions and set aside.

2. In a saucepan over medium heat, combine the coconut milk, water, tamari, rice vinegar, salt, and pepper. Add the chicken and bring to a simmer for 10 minutes or cooked through.

3. Stir in the spinach and remove from heat. When the spinach has wilted, divide into bowls along with the rice and enjoy!

NUTRITION - AMOUNT PER SERVING

Calories	527	Sugar	2g
Fat	24g	Protein	33g
Carbs	44g	Cholesterol	82mg
Fiber	2g	Sodium	632mg

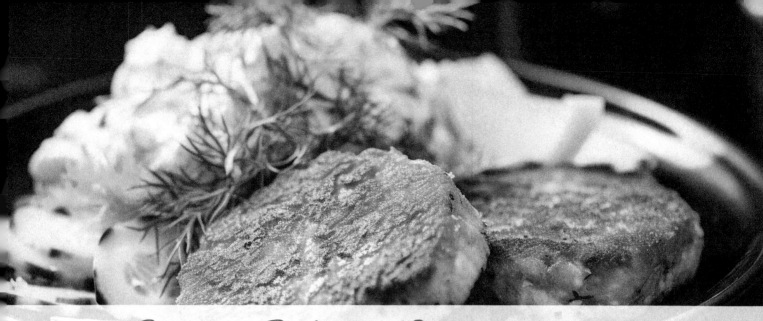

Ginger Salmon Patties with Fennel & Cucumber Salad

 20 Minutes

 1 Serving

INGREDIENTS

- 1 1/4 tbsps Extra Virgin Olive Oil (divided)
- 1 1/2 tsps Lime Juice
- 1/2 tsp Maple Syrup
- 1/8 tsp Sea Salt (divided)
- 1/2 Cucumber (large, thinly sliced)
- 1/2 bulb Fennel (small, thinly sliced)
- 2 tbsps Fresh Dill (chopped)
- 170 grams Salmon Fillet (skinless, chopped into small chunks)
- 1 1/2 tsps Ginger (grated)

INSTRUCTIONS

1. In a medium bowl, whisk together ⅗ of the oil, the lime juice, maple syrup, and half of the sea salt. Add the cucumber, fennel, and dill and toss to coat.

2. In a separate bowl, add the salmon chunks, ginger, and the remaining salt. Mix gently.

3. Divide the salmon mixture evenly into equal parts, and form into slightly flattened patties, about 3 to 4 inches in diameter.

4. Add the remaining oil to a non-stick pan over medium heat. Cook the patties for 6 to 8 minutes , flipping once halfway.

5. Serve the salad and salmon patties on a plate and enjoy!

NUTRITION - AMOUNT PER SERVING

Calories	444	Sugar	9g
Fat	25g	Protein	40g
Carbs	17g	Cholesterol	87mg
Fiber	4g	Sodium	493mg

Dinners

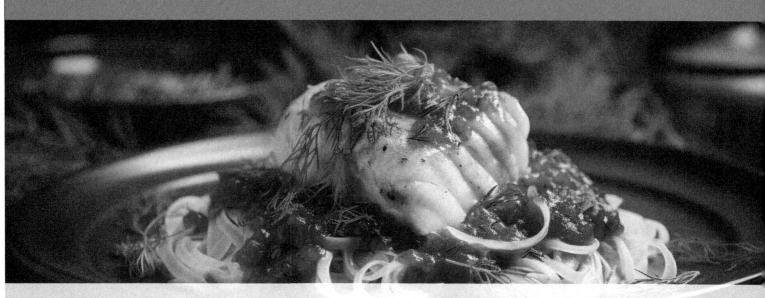

Poached Cod in Tomato Sauce with Spaghetti

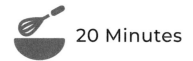 20 Minutes

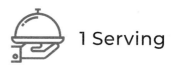 1 Serving

INGREDIENTS

- 1/4 cup Brown Rice Spaghetti
- 3/4 cup Tomato Sauce
- Sea Salt & Black Pepper (to taste)
- 1 Cod Fillet
- 1/4 Lemon (juiced)
- 1 tbsp Fresh Dill

INSTRUCTIONS

1. Cook the spaghetti according to the directions on the package.
2. Meanwhile, in a pan with a lid add the tomato sauce and simmer gently. Season with salt and pepper to taste.
3. Place the cod fillets in the tomato sauce, close the pan with a lid, and let them simmer for about 15 minutes or until cooked through.
4. Plate the spaghetti before topping with fish and tomato sauce. Squeeze the lemon juice over the top and sprinkle with dill for extra flavor.

NUTRITION - AMOUNT PER SERVING

Calories	436	Sugar	7g
Fat	4g	Protein	47g
Carbs	54g	Cholesterol	99mg
Fiber	5g	Sodium	145mg

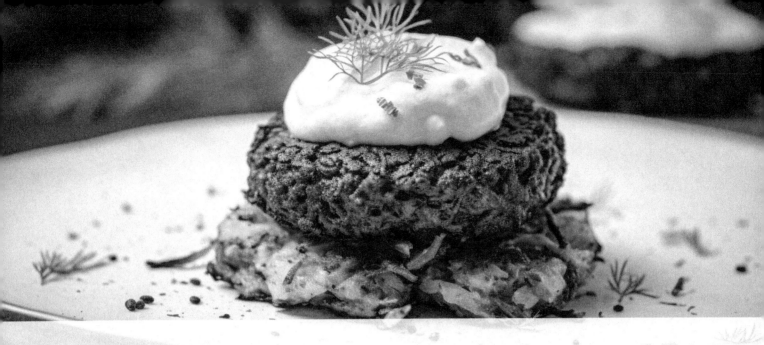

Celery Root Latkes & Beef Patties

 10 Minutes

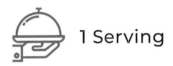 1 Serving

INGREDIENTS

- 1 cup Celery Root (shredded)
- 1/2 Egg
- 1/8 tsp Dried Dill
- Sea Salt & Black Pepper (to taste)
- 1/2 tsp Extra Virgin Olive Oil (divided)
- 113 grams Lean Ground Beef
- 1 1/3 tbsps Unsweetened Coconut Yogurt

INSTRUCTIONS

1. In a large bowl, combine the shredded celery root, egg, dill, salt, and pepper. Mix until well combined.

2. Use half the oil in a large pan and heat over medium heat. Form the celery root mixture into patties with your hands, about ½ cup per latke. Transfer to the frying pan and cook for 5 minutes on each side or until golden.

3. Form the ground beef into even patties, approximately 3 to 4 inches in diameter. Then, in the same pan, use the rest of the extra virgin olive oil. Once warm, add the beef patties. Cook for 5 to 6 minutes on each side or until cooked through.

4. Serve the beef patties on top of the latkes. Top with coconut yogurt and enjoy!

NUTRITION - AMOUNT PER SERVING

Calories	419	Sugar	3g
Fat	28g	Protein	25g
Carbs	16g	Cholesterol	174mg
Fiber	3g	Sodium	271mg

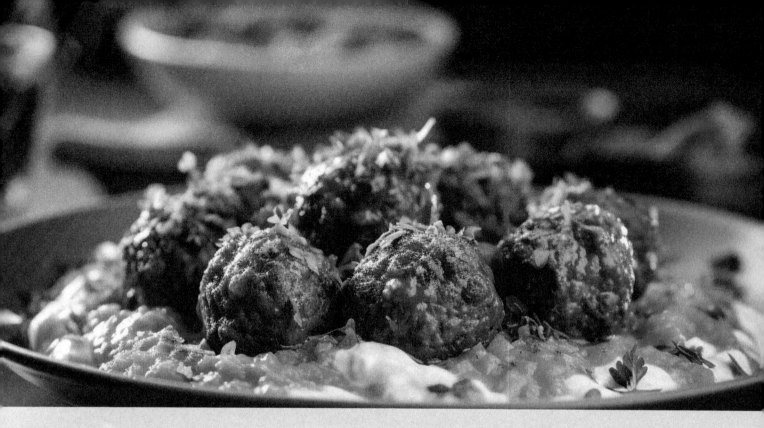

Meatballs & Carrot Mash

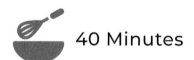 40 Minutes

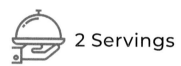 2 Servings

INGREDIENTS

- 213 grams Extra Lean Ground Beef
- Sea Salt & Black Pepper (to taste)
- 4 Carrots (medium, peeled, diced)
- 1 1/2 tsps Butter
- 2 tbsps Mint Leaves
- 1/2 Lime (cut into wedges)

INSTRUCTIONS

1. Preheat the oven to 400°F (205°C) and prepare a baking sheet covered with parchment paper.

2. Mix the ground beef, salt, and pepper together in a large bowl. Roll the beef into one-inch balls and place them on the baking sheet. Bake for 20 to 25 minutes or until cooked through.

3. Meanwhile, add the carrots to a pot and cover with water. Bring to a boil and cook for ten minutes or until the carrots are tender. Drain the water, add butter to the carrots, and mash everything together.

4. Divide the carrot mash and meatballs between serving plates. Top with mint leaves and lime juice.

NUTRITION - AMOUNT PER SERVING

Calories	266	Sugar	6g
Fat	14g	Protein	23g
Carbs	13g	Cholesterol	77mg
Fiber	4g	Sodium	155mg

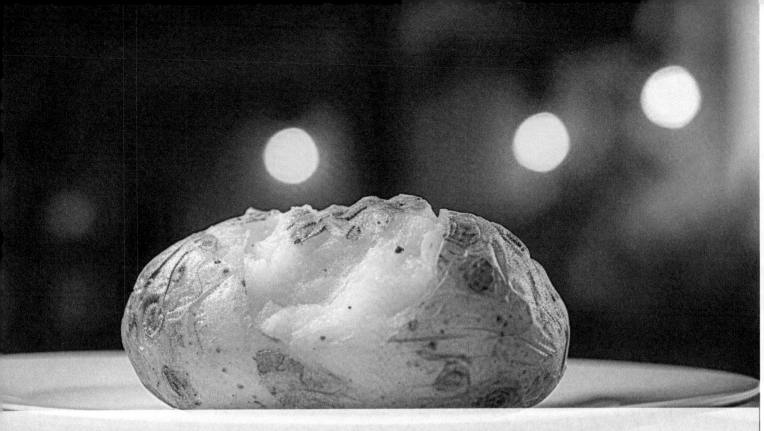

Baked Potato

 45 Minutes

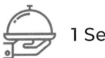 1 Serving

INGREDIENTS

- 1 Russet Potato (large)
- 1/4 tsp Extra Virgin Olive Oil (optional)
- 1/16 tsp Sea Salt (optional)

INSTRUCTIONS

1. Preheat oven to 400°F (204°C). Scrub the potato and pierce it multiple times with a fork.

2. Lightly coat the potato in olive oil and season with sea salt (optional). Place the potato on a baking sheet and bake in the oven for about 45 to 50 minutes until thoroughly cooked and tender.

3. To serve, cut lengthwise down the center of the potato before carefully squeezing the ends together to open.

NUTRITION - AMOUNT PER SERVING

Calories	174	Sugar	2g
Fat	1g	Protein	5g
Carbs	37g	Cholesterol	0mg
Fiber	4g	Sodium	172mg

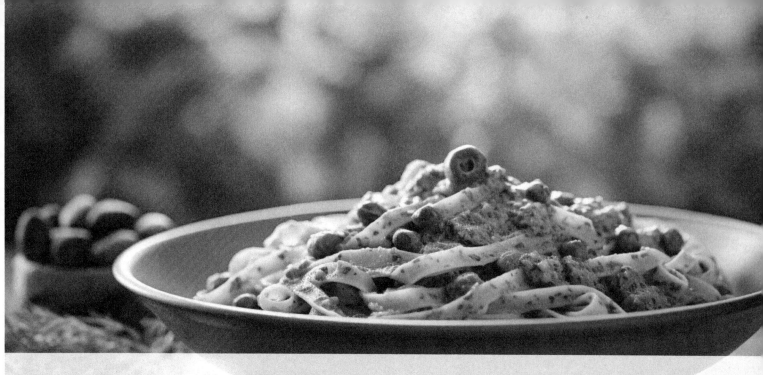

Mediterranean Pasta with Kale

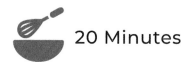 20 Minutes

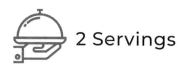 2 Servings

INGREDIENTS

- 113 grams Brown Rice Fettuccine
- 2 cups Kale Leaves (finely chopped)
- 1/4 cup Pitted Kalamata Olives
- 1 tbsp Lemon Juice
- 2 tbsps Extra Virgin Olive Oil
- 1 tbsp Nutritional Yeast
- 1/8 tsp Sea Salt

INSTRUCTIONS

1. Prepare the pasta following the packaging instructions. Once the pasta is cooked and strained, rinse it with cold water to prevent overcooking. Set it aside.

2. In the same pot used for the pasta, add the kale and olives and cook over low-medium heat for about 3 to 4 minutes, until the kale is soft.

3. Return the pasta to the pot along with the lemon juice, extra virgin olive oil, nutritional yeast, and sea salt. Toss to combine.

4. Divide onto plates and enjoy!

NUTRITION - AMOUNT PER SERVING

Calories	371	Sugar	1g
Fat	18g	Protein	7g
Carbs	47g	Cholesterol	0mg
Fiber	5g	Sodium	295mg

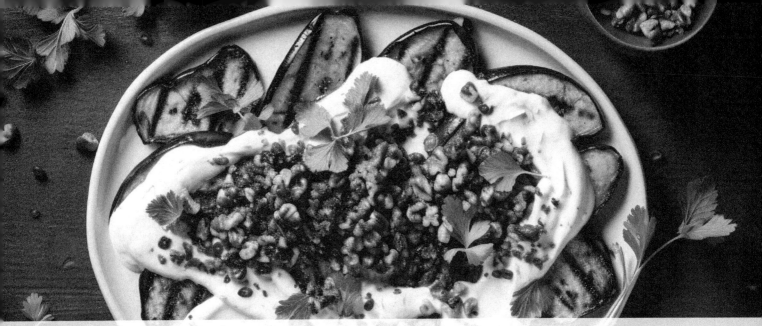

Grilled Eggplant with Spiced Walnuts & Yogurt

 25 Minutes

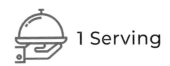 1 Serving

INGREDIENTS

- 75 grams Eggplant (small, cut in half lengthwise)
- 1 1/2 tsps Avocado Oil (divided)
- 3/4 tsp Cumin (divided)
- Sea Salt & Black Pepper (to taste)
- 30 grams Walnuts (chopped)
- 1 1/2 tsps Coconut Aminos
- 1/4 cup Unsweetened Coconut Yogurt
- 1 tbsp Cilantro (chopped)

INSTRUCTIONS

1. Score the flesh of the eggplant and brush with half of the oil. Season with half of the cumin, salt, and pepper.

2. Heat the grill or a grill pan to medium-high heat. Once hot, place the eggplant on the grill, flesh side down. Grill for 5 minutes on each side until golden brown and soft to the touch. Set aside.

3. In a small frying pan, on medium-low heat, toast the walnuts with the remaining oil, coconut aminos, and the remaining cumin for about 3 minutes. Remove from heat and set aside.

4. To assemble, top the eggplant with equal parts of yogurt, walnuts, and cilantro.

NUTRITION - AMOUNT PER SERVING

Calories	316	Sugar	5g
Fat	29g	Protein	6g
Carbs	14g	Cholesterol	0mg
Fiber	5g	Sodium	153mg

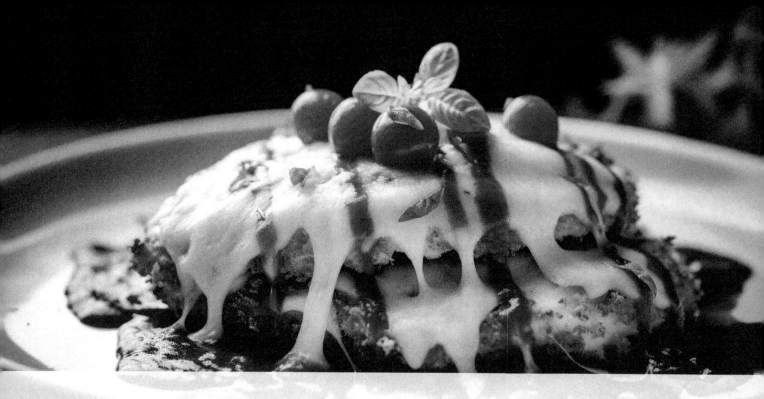

Baked Pizza Chicken

 25 Minutes

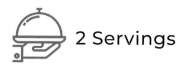 2 Servings

INGREDIENTS

- 227 grams Chicken Breast
- 1/2 tsp Italian Seasoning
- Sea Salt & Black Pepper (to taste)
- 2 tbsps Tomato Sauce
- 28 grams Mozzarella Cheese (shredded)

INSTRUCTIONS

1. Heat the oven to 400°F (205°C) and line a baking sheet with parchment paper.

2. Slice the chicken breast(s) lengthwise to create cutlets. Arrange the chicken cutlets on the baking sheet and season both sides with Italian seasoning, sea salt, and black pepper to your taste. Bake for about 12 to 15 minutes until the chicken is fully cooked.

3. Take the baking sheet from the oven carefully and adjust the oven setting to broil.

4. Top the chicken cutlets evenly with the tomato sauce and cheese. Broil for 1 to 2 minutes or until the cheese has melted.

5. Divide evenly between plates or on-the-go containers and enjoy!

NUTRITION - AMOUNT PER SERVING

Calories	175	Sugar	1g
Fat	6g	Protein	28g
Carbs	1g	Cholesterol	95mg
Fiber	0g	Sodium	98mg

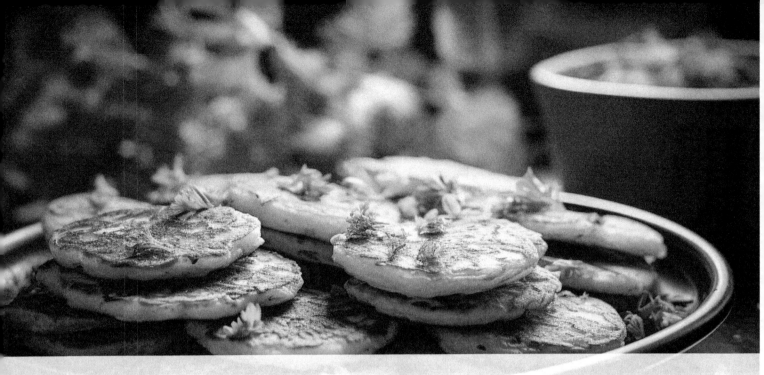

Potato Patties

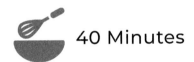 **40 Minutes**

 **1 Serving**

INGREDIENTS

- 1/2 cup Water
- 1/2 Russet Potato (peeled, chopped)
- 1 tbsp Unsweetened Almond Milk
- 1 1/2 tsps Avocado Oil (divided)
- 1/16 tsp Sea Salt
- 1/16 tsp Black Pepper
- 3/4 tsp Parsley (chopped)

INSTRUCTIONS

1. Bring a small saucepan of water to a boil and then add the chopped potatoes to the boiling water and cook until soft for about 10 to 12 minutes. After cooking the potatoes, drain the water and add the almond milk, half of the avocado oil, sea salt, and pepper. Use a potato masher to blend everything until it's smooth.

2. Add the remaining avocado oil to a skillet and heat over medium heat. Take ½ cup of the mashed potatoes and press them down with a spatula to create a pancake shape. Cook each side for 8 to 10 minutes or until they turn a lovely golden brown. Repeat this process until all the mashed potatoes are cooked.

3. To serve plate and top with parsley.

NUTRITION - AMOUNT PER SERVING

Calories	147	Sugar	1g
Fat	7g	Protein	2g
Carbs	19g	Cholesterol	0mg
Fiber	2g	Sodium	173mg

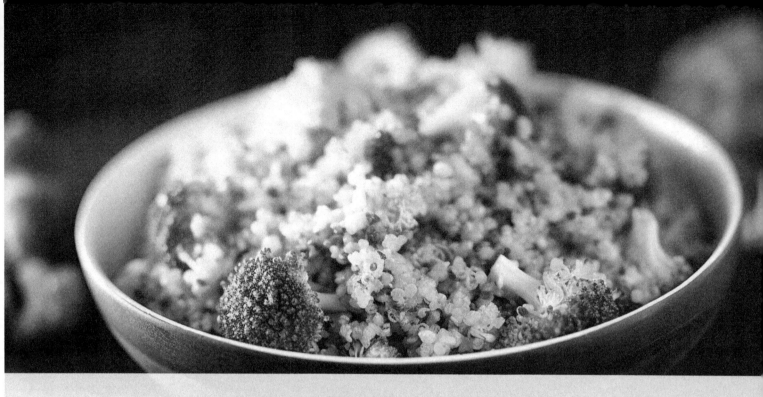

Cheezy Broccoli Quinoa

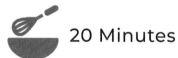 20 Minutes

 3 Servings

INGREDIENTS

- 3/4 cup Quinoa (uncooked)
- 1 1/3 cups Water
- 75 grams Broccoli Florets
- 2 1/4 tsps Nutritional Yeast
- Sea Salt & Black Pepper (to taste)

INSTRUCTIONS

1. Following packaging instructions, add the quinoa and water to a small pot. On high heat, bring the pot ingredients to a boil, then reduce to a simmer for about 12 to 15 minutes until all water is absorbed. Fluff with a fork and set aside.

2. While the quinoa cooks, lightly steam the broccoli florets. Once tender, drain the water then chop coarsely.

3. Mix the quinoa, broccoli, and nutritional yeast together. To taste, season with sea salt and black pepper. Toss well to mix and enjoy!

NUTRITION - AMOUNT PER SERVING

Calories	173	Sugar	0g
Fat	3g	Protein	8g
Carbs	30g	Cholesterol	0mg
Fiber	4g	Sodium	19mg

Snacks

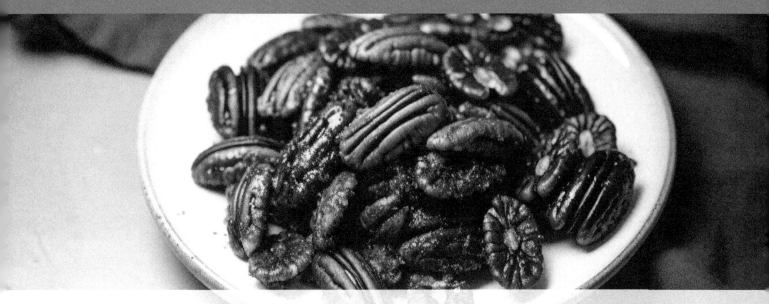

Sweet & Spicy Candied Pecans

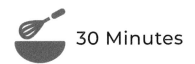 30 Minutes

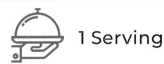 1 Serving

INGREDIENTS

- 1/4 cup Pecans
- 3/4 tsp Maple Syrup
- 1/16 tsp Cinnamon
- 1/16 tsp Cayenne Pepper
- 1/16 tsp Sea Salt

INSTRUCTIONS

1. Preheat the oven to 350°F (175°C) and line a baking sheet with parchment paper.

2. In a small bowl, toss together all ingredients, then transfer to the baking sheet. Spread across the baking sheet evenly. Bake for 5 to 7 minutes, flip the pecans or stir and then bake for 7 minutes more.

3. Remove the baking sheet from the oven and let the pecans rest for 15 minutes before serving.

NUTRITION - AMOUNT PER SERVING

Calories	185	Sugar	4g
Fat	18g	Protein	2g
Carbs	7g	Cholesterol	0mg
Fiber	2g	Sodium	148mg

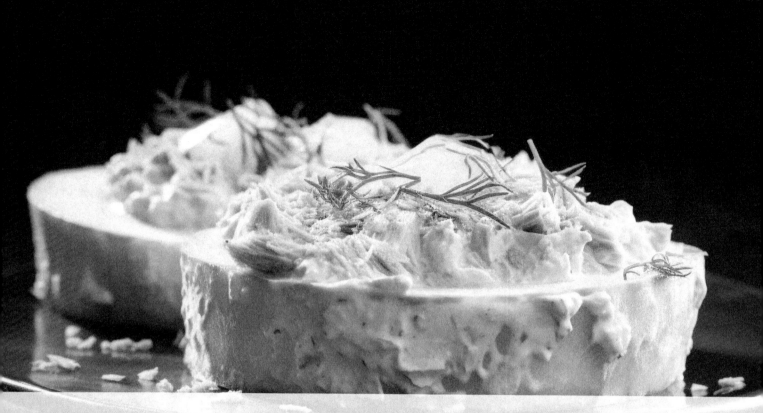

Cucumber Tuna Bites

 5 Minutes

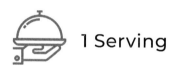 1 Serving

INGREDIENTS

- ½ can Tuna (flaked and drained)
- 1 tbsp Cream Cheese (regular)
- ½ Cucumber (large, sliced into rounds)

INSTRUCTIONS

1. Add the tuna to a small bowl with the cream cheese and mix together.
2. Top each cucumber round with a spoonful of the tuna mixture.

NUTRITION - AMOUNT PER SERVING

Calories	138	Sugar	3g
Fat	5g	Protein	18g
Carbs	6g	Cholesterol	43mg
Fiber	1g	Sodium	272mg

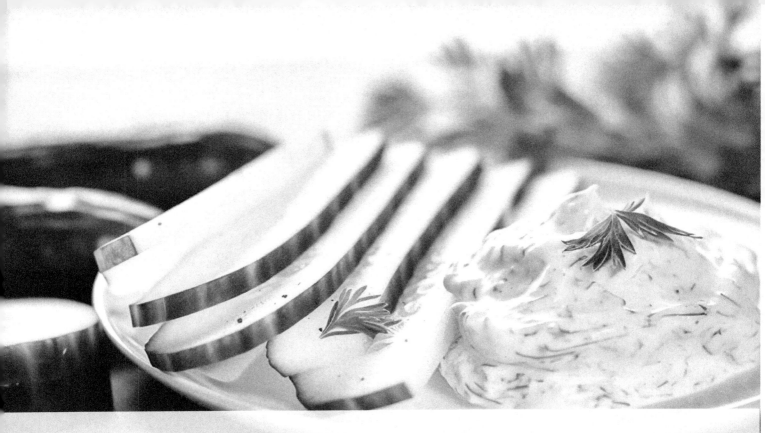

Cucumber & Herbed Yogurt Dip

 5 Minutes

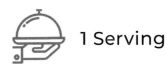 1 Serving

INGREDIENTS

- 1/3 cup Unsweetened Coconut Yogurt
- 1 tbsp Fresh Dill (finely chopped)
- 1 tbsp Parsley (finely chopped)
- 1/4 tsp Sea Salt (to taste)
- 1/2 Cucumber (large, sliced)

INSTRUCTIONS

1. In a bowl, combine the coconut yogurt, dill, parsley, and salt.
2. Serve alongside the cucumber slices.

NUTRITION - AMOUNT PER SERVING

Calories	61	Sugar	3g
Fat	3g	Protein	1g
Carbs	10g	Cholesterol	0mg
Fiber	2g	Sodium	612mg

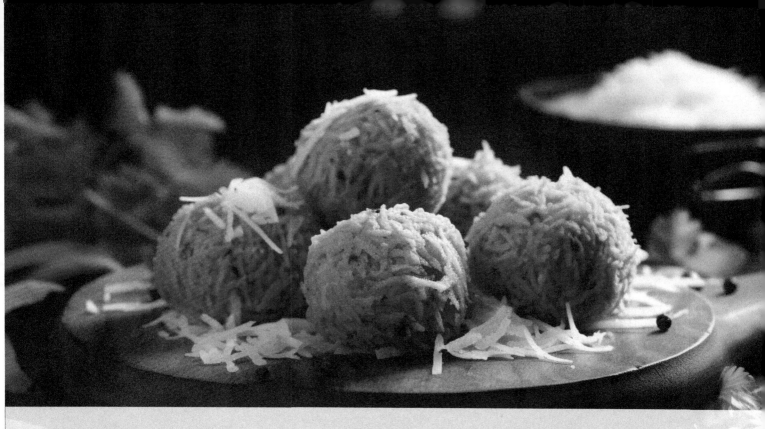

Cheese & Carrot Balls

 5 Minutes

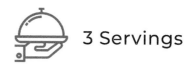 3 Servings

INGREDIENTS

- 2 Carrots (medium, grated)
- 113 grams Cheddar Cheese (shredded)

INSTRUCTIONS

1. Add the carrot and cheese to a bowl and mix to combine.
2. Form into even balls with your hands, roughly one inch in diameter.
3. Serve on a plate and enjoy.

NUTRITION - AMOUNT PER SERVING

Calories	169	Sugar	2g
Fat	13g	Protein	9g
Carbs	5g	Cholesterol	37mg
Fiber	1g	Sodium	275mg

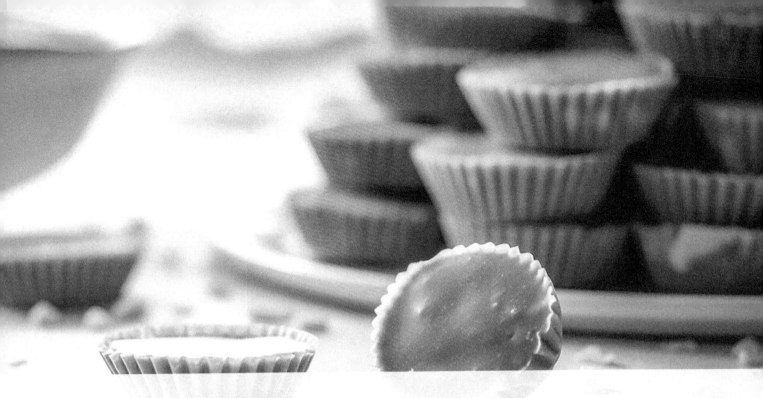

Salted Peanut Fat Bombs

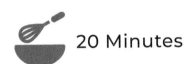 20 Minutes

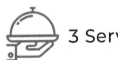 3 Servings

INGREDIENTS

- 1/4 cup All Natural Peanut Butter
- 2 tbsps Coconut Oil
- 1/8 tsp Sea Salt
- 1/16 tsp Stevia Powder

INSTRUCTIONS

1. Arrange the paper baking cups on a plate or baking sheet and set aside.
2. Prepare a double boiler by filling a medium pot with about an inch of water. Place a smaller pot or a heat-safe bowl on top, making sure the water does not touch the smaller pot or bowl. Ensure that the smaller pot or bowl sits securely on top of the larger pot and that no water or steam can escape. Bring the water to a boil and then reduce the heat to the lowest setting.
3. Place the coconut oil and peanut butter in the smaller pot. Let them melt and then stir to blend before mixing in the stevia powder and salt.
4. Divide the peanut butter mixture among the paper baking cups, then place them in the freezer. Let the fat bombs set for a minimum of 30 minutes until they become solid. Remove from the paper cups and transfer them to a suitable container to store in the freezer.

NUTRITION - AMOUNT PER SERVING

Calories	209	Sugar	2g
Fat	20g	Protein	5g
Carbs	5g	Cholesterol	0mg
Fiber	1g	Sodium	102mg

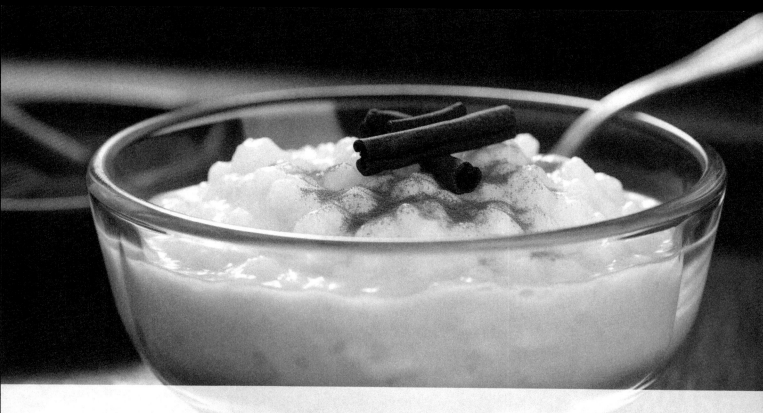

Vanilla Rice Pudding

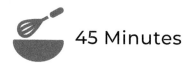 45 Minutes

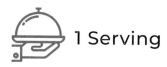 1 Serving

INGREDIENTS

- 1 cup Unsweetened Almond Milk
- 1 1/3 tbsps Maple Syrup
- 2/3 tsp Vanilla Extract
- 1/16 tsp Sea Salt
- 2 2/3 tbsps Arborio Rice

INSTRUCTIONS

1. In a large pot, mix the almond milk, maple syrup, vanilla, and sea salt together. Heat the almond milk mixture over a medium heat until it reaches a gentle boil before adding the rice. Reduce the heat to low.

2. Let the rice gently simmer, stirring frequently. It's best to stir every 3 to 5 minutes to avoid sticking and to assist in thickening the pudding. Keep this up for about 20 to 25 minutes, or until the rice becomes tender, the liquid is absorbed, and the pudding reaches the desired thickness.

3. Take off the heat and allow the rice pudding to cool in the pot for 10 minutes. During this time, it will continue to thicken.

NUTRITION - AMOUNT PER SERVING

Calories	226	Sugar	16g
Fat	3g	Protein	3g
Carbs	47g	Cholesterol	0mg
Fiber	1g	Sodium	263mg

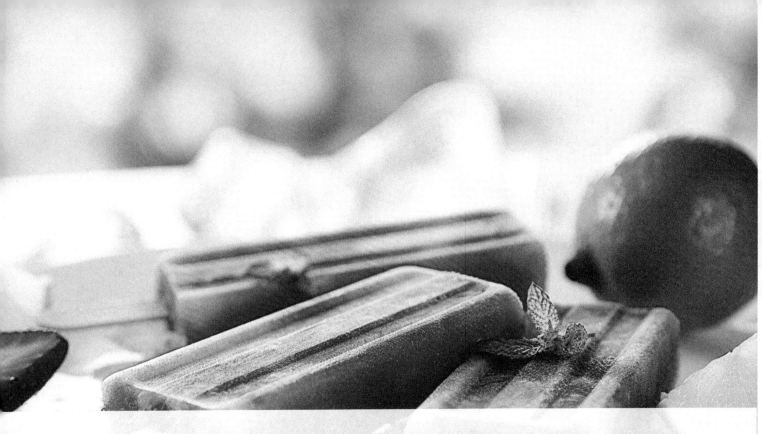

Strawberry Lime Popsicles

 6 Hours

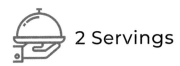 2 Servings

INGREDIENTS

- 65 grams Strawberries (stems removed)
- 1/3 Lime (large, juiced)
- 2 tsps Maple Syrup
- 1 tsp Chia Seeds

INSTRUCTIONS

1. Blend all the required ingredients in a blender until the mixture is smooth in texture.

2. Pour the popsicle mixture into the popsicle molds and freeze for 5 to 6 hours until completely frozen.

NUTRITION - AMOUNT PER SERVING

Calories	39	Sugar	6g
Fat	1g	Protein	1g
Carbs	8g	Cholesterol	0mg
Fiber	1g	Sodium	2mg

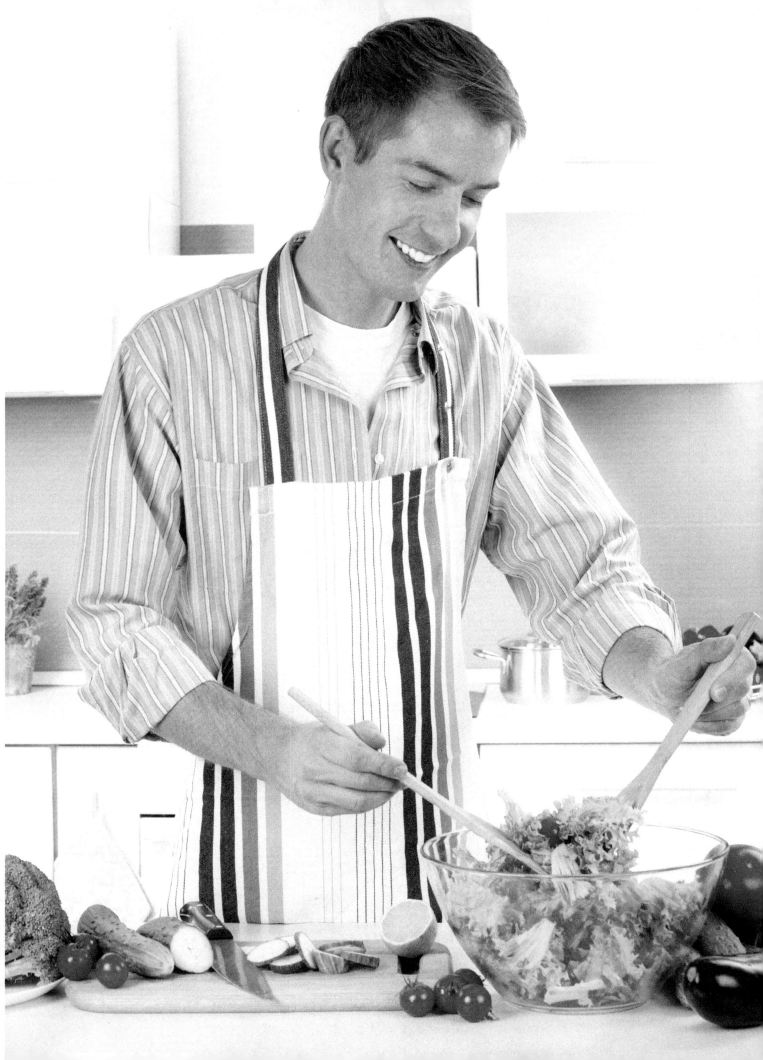

WEEK 2

7-Days Meal Plan

MONDAY

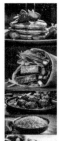

BREAKFAST
Strawberry Buckwheat Pancakes

LUNCH
Tofu Veggie Wrap

DINNER
Beef Meatballs, Brown Rice

SNACKS
Macadamia Nut Clusters

TUESDAY

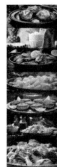

BREAKFAST
Tuna & Goat Cheese Egg Muffns, Pineapple Cucumber Smoothie

LUNCH
Air Fryer Lemon Dill Chicken Wings, Boiled Potato

DINNER
Mackerel Fish Cakes, Mashed Carrots

SNACKS
Creamy Spiced Broccoli

WEDNESDAY

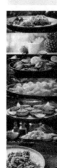

BREAKFAST
Tomato & Brie Omelet, Pineapple Lime Smoothie

LUNCH
Lemon & Cilantro Baked Pickerel, Brown Rice

DINNER
One Pan Roasted Tahini Chicken & Potato

SNACKS
Cheezy Walnuts

THURSDAY

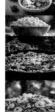

BREAKFAST
Cinnamon Maple Brown Rice Porridge, Macadamia Nuts

LUNCH
One Pot Cheeseburger Pasta

DINNER
Shrimp, Kale & Quinoa Salad

SNACKS
Pineapple Chia Pudding

FRIDAY

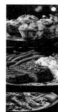

BREAKFAST
Kale & Mozzarella Egg Muffns

LUNCH
Steak, Mashed Potatoes & Green Beans

DINNER
Coconut Yogurt Chicken, Crispy Eggplant Fries

SNACKS
Radish & Cucumber Rice Cakes

SATURDAY

BREAKFAST
Egg in a Hole, Strawberry Orange Smoothie

LUNCH
Coconut Cod & Spinach with Rice

DINNER
Chicken & Quinoa Meatballs, Pan Fried Zucchini

SNACKS
Sea Salted Coconut Kale Chips

SUNDAY

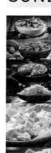

BREAKFAST
Coconut Chia Seed Yogurt, Toasted Walnuts

LUNCH
Roasted Potato Frittata, Carrot Salad

DINNER
Creamy Herb Chicken Lettuce Wraps

SNACKS
Tropical Fruit Salad

Shopping List

FRUITS
1 Kiwi
2 ¹⁄₁₆ Lemon
1 ½ tsps Lemon Juice
1 Lime
1 Navel Orange
1 cup Papaya
2 ¾ cups Pineapple
½ cup Strawberries
60 grams Strawberries

SEEDS, NUTS & SPICES
1 Bay Leaf
¼ tsp Cardamom
⅓ cup Chia Seeds
1 tbsp Cinnamon
2 tsps Cumin
1 ¼ tsps Curry Powder
⅓ tsp Dried Basil
⅓ tsp Italian Seasoning
½ cup Macadamia Nuts
Sea Salt & Black Pepper
½ cup Walnuts

FROZEN
½ cup Frozen Strawberries
3 Ice Cubes

VEGETABLES
5 ⅔ cups Baby Spinach
65 grams Broccoli
11 ⅔ Carrots
½ cup Cherry Tomatoes
⅓ cup Cilantro
1 ¼ Cucumber
⅓ Eggplant
¼ cup Fresh Dill
1 ½ tsps Ginger
75 grams Green Beans
⅛ head Green Lettuce
3 cups Kale Leaves
1 tbsp Mint Leaves

⅓ cup Parsley
1 cup Purple Cabbage
½ cup Radishes
4 Yellow Potatoes
75 grams Zucchini

PANTRY STAPLES
1 ⅓ cups Brown Rice
½ cup Brown Rice Macaroni
¾ cup Canned Coconut Milk
½ cup Diced Tomatoes
¼ cup Jasmine Rice
⅓ cup Quinoa
½ can Tuna
4 Brown Rice Cake
⅓ cup Maple Syrup
½ cup Rice Puffs Cereal
2 Brown Rice Tortillas

BAKING
½ tsp Baking Powder
1 tbsp Brown Rice Flour
½ cup Buckwheat Flour
½ tsp Coconut Sugar
⅓ cup Cornmeal
19 grams Dark Chocolate
½ tsp Nutritional Yeast
1 ½ tsps Vanilla Extract

BREAD, FISH, MEAT & CHEESE
56 grams Brie Cheese
76 grams Canned Mackerel
19 grams Cheddar Cheese
113 grams Chicken Breast
227 grams Chicken Breast, Cooked
227 grams Chicken Thighs
340 grams Chicken Wings
1 Cod Fillet
339 grams Extra Lean Ground Beef

227 grams Extra Lean Ground Chicken
2 slices Gluten-free Bread
1 ½ tbsps Goat Cheese
50 grams Mozzarella Cheese
142 grams Pickerel Fillet
227 grams Shrimp
282 grams Tofu
113 grams Top Sirloin Steak

CONDIMENTS & OILS
1 ⅛ tbsps Apple Cider Vinegar
1 ¾ tbsps Avocado Oil
2 grams Avocado Oil Spray
2 ¾ tbsps Coconut Oil
⅓ cup Extra Virgin Olive Oil
1 tsp Fish Sauce
1 ½ tsps Rice Vinegar
1 ½ tsps Tahini
2 ½ tbsps Tamari

FRIDGE
3 ⅛ tbsps Butter
19 Eggs
59 milliliters Pineapple Juice
1 cup Plain Coconut Milk
3 ¼ cups Unsweetened Almond Milk
2 ¹⁄₁₆ cups Unsweetened Coconut Yogurt

Breakfasts

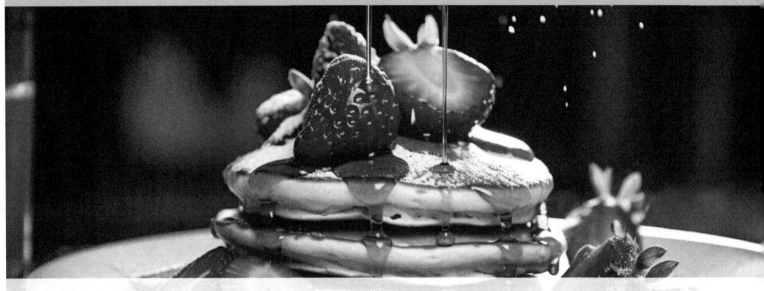

Strawberry Buckwheat Pancakes

 10 Minutes

 1 Serving

INGREDIENTS

- 1/2 cup Buckwheat Flour
- 1/2 cup Unsweetened Almond Milk
- 1 1/2 tsps Coconut Oil (melted)
- 1 1/2 tbsps Maple Syrup (divided)
- 1/2 tsp Baking Powder
- 1/2 tsp Vanilla Extract
- 1/2 Egg (whisked)
- 1/4 cup Strawberries (sliced)

INSTRUCTIONS

1. In a large bowl, whisk together the buckwheat flour, milk, coconut oil, 1/3 of the maple syrup, baking powder, vanilla extract, and egg.

2. Heat a non-stick pan over medium heat, and add 1/4 cup of the pancake batter. Flip after the batter starts to bubble, about 2 to 3 minutes, and cook for an additional 2 to 3 minutes. Repeat with the remaining batter.

3. Serve the pancakes with sliced strawberries and remaining maple syrup.

NUTRITION - AMOUNT PER SERVING

Calories	407	Sugar	20g
Fat	12g	Protein	12g
Carbs	66g	Cholesterol	93mg
Fiber	9g	Sodium	364mg

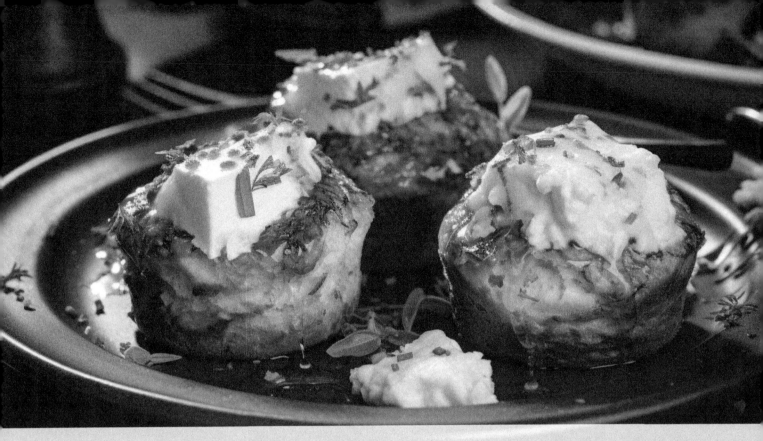

Tuna & Goat Cheese Egg Muffins

 35 Minutes

 5 Servings

INGREDIENTS

- 1 ½ Egg (large, whisked)
- 2 tbsps Unsweetened Almond Milk
- ½ can Tuna (drained, flaked)
- 1 ½ tbsps Goat Cheese
- ⅛ tsp Black Pepper

INSTRUCTIONS

1. Preheat the oven to 375°F (190°C). Prepare a muffin tray by lining it with paper baking cups or use a silicone muffin tray.

2. Add the eggs, almond milk, and tuna to a bowl. Mix until well combined. Divide the mixture evenly between muffin cups. Top with goat cheese and season with black pepper.

3. Bake in the oven for about 25 minutes until firm.

NUTRITION - AMOUNT PER SERVING

Calories	42	Sugar	0g
Fat	2g	Protein	5g
Carbs	0g	Cholesterol	62mg
Fiber	0g	Sodium	76mg

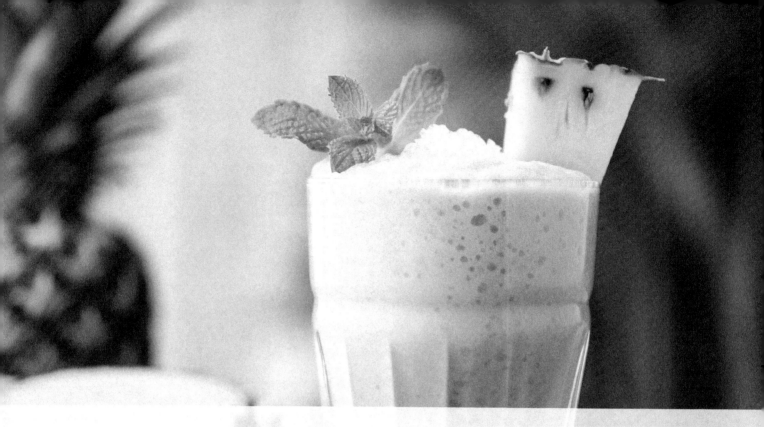

Pineapple Cucumber Smoothie

 2 Minutes

 1 Serving

INGREDIENTS

- 1 cup Pineapple (fresh or frozen)
- 1 cup Baby Spinach
- 1/2 cup Water
- 1/4 Cucumber (roughly chopped)
- 1 1/2 tsps Lemon Juice
- 1 1/2 tsps Chia Seeds (optional)
- 1 tsp Ginger (fresh, grated, optional)

INSTRUCTIONS

1. Place all the ingredients into a blender and blend until the mixture is smooth.

2. Pour into a glass to enjoy your smoothie.

NUTRITION - AMOUNT PER SERVING

Calories	132	Sugar	18g
Fat	2g	Protein	3g
Carbs	29g	Cholesterol	0mg
Fiber	5g	Sodium	30mg

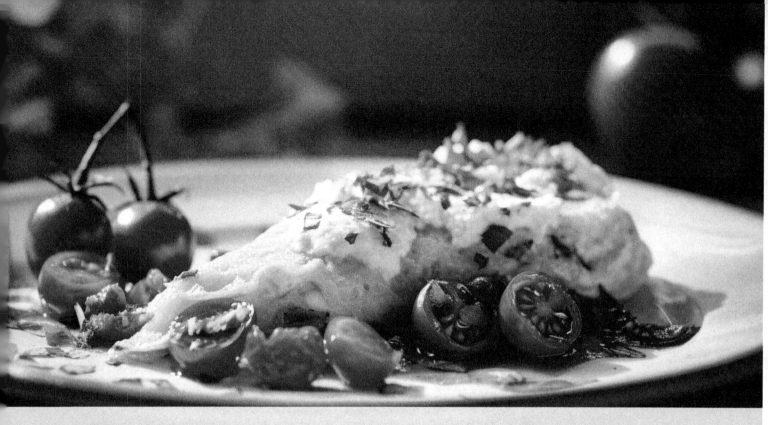

Tomato & Brie Omelet

 15 Minutes

 2 Servings

INGREDIENTS

- 2 tsps Butter
- 4 Eggs
- 2 tbsps Parsley (chopped)
- Sea Salt & Black Pepper (to taste)
- 56 grams Brie Cheese
- ½ cup Cherry Tomatoes (halved)

INSTRUCTIONS

1. In a small non-stick pan, melt the butter over medium heat.

2. Beat the eggs and parsley in a bowl. Season with sea salt and pepper before pouring the egg mixture into the pan. Cook until the eggs are nearly set. Next, place the brie and tomatoes on one half of the omelet and fold the other half over the top.

3. Remove from heat, serve on a plate, and enjoy!

NUTRITION - AMOUNT PER SERVING

Calories	280	Sugar	2g
Fat	21g	Protein	19g
Carbs	3g	Cholesterol	411mg
Fiber	1g	Sodium	325mg

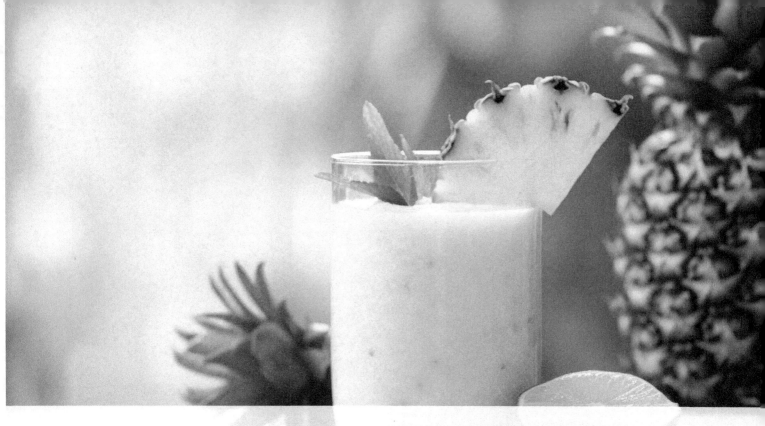

Pineapple Lime Smoothie

 5 Minutes

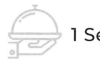 1 Serving

INGREDIENTS

- 2/3 cup Unsweetened Almond Milk
- 2/3 cup Pineapple
- 1 tbsp Maple Syrup
- 3 Ice Cubes
- 1/2 Lime (juiced, zested)

INSTRUCTIONS

1. Add all ingredients to a blender except for the lime juice and zest. Blend until smooth.
2. Add the lime juice and zest, and pulse two to three more times. Serve immediately and enjoy!

NUTRITION - AMOUNT PER SERVING

Calories	132	Sugar	23g
Fat	2g	Protein	1g
Carbs	30g	Cholesterol	0mg
Fiber	2g	Sodium	111mg

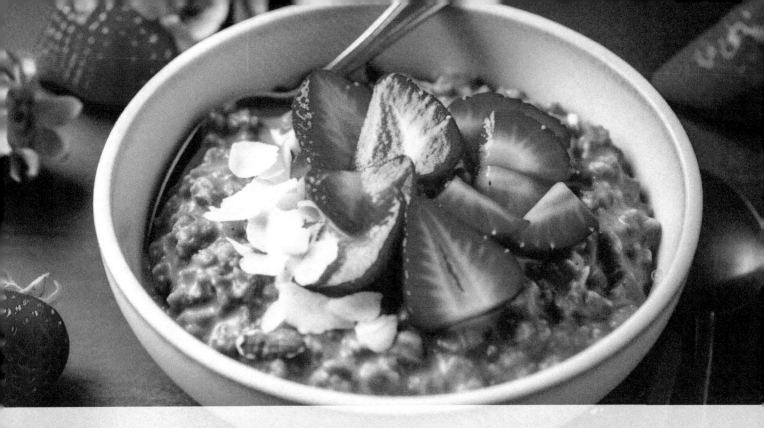

Cinnamon Maple Brown Rice Porridge

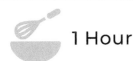 1 Hour

 2 Servings

INGREDIENTS

- 2 cups Unsweetened Almond Milk
- 2 tbsps Maple Syrup
- 1½ tsps Cinnamon
- 1 tsp Vanilla Extract
- ½ cup Brown Rice (long grain, rinsed well under cold water)
- 60 grams Strawberries (chopped)

INSTRUCTIONS

1. Add the almond milk, maple syrup, cinnamon and vanilla to a large saucepan with a tight-fitting lid. Bring to a gentle boil then stir in the rice.

2. Reduce heat to low and cover the pot with the lid. Let it cook, stirring occasionally, for 50 to 55 minutes, or until the rice is very tender and the porridge has thickened.

3. Divide the porridge between bowls and top with the chopped strawberries. Serve with additional almond milk, maple syrup and cinnamon if desired and enjoy!

NUTRITION - AMOUNT PER SERVING

Calories	271	Sugar	14g
Fat	4g	Protein	5g
Carbs	54g	Cholesterol	0mg
Fiber	4g	Sodium	166mg

REFER TO PAGE 45 FOR THE ACCOMPANYING MACADAMIA NUTS RECIPE

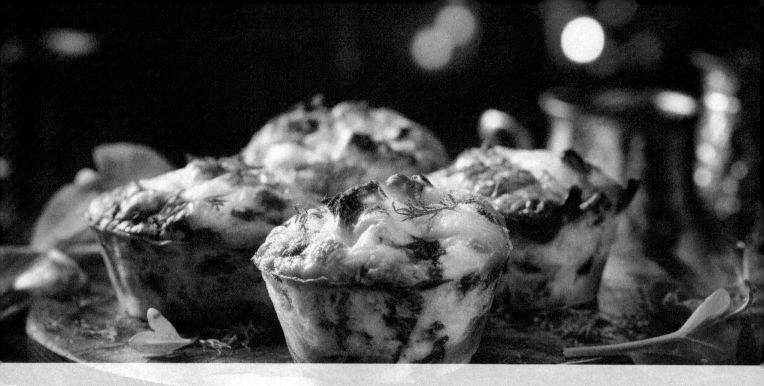

Kale & Mozzarella Egg Muffins

 25 Minutes

 3 Servings

INGREDIENTS

- 1 tbsp Extra Virgin Olive Oil (divided)
- 50 grams Mozzarella Cheese (thinly sliced, chopped)
- 1 cup Kale Leaves (finely chopped)
- 4 Eggs
- 2 tbsps Water
- Sea Salt & Black Pepper (to taste)

INSTRUCTIONS

1. Heat the oven to 375°F (190°C). Use a silicone muffin tray or prepare a muffin tray by lining it with paper baking cups.

2. Pour the oil into the pan, then add the kale leaves. Cook for 2 to 3 minutes until the kale leaves become wilted and tender. Sprinkle the cheese onto the kale and stir everything together.

3. Divide the kale and cheese between the cups of the prepared muffin tray.

4. Add the eggs and water to a small bowl and whisk well. Pour the eggs into the prepared tray. Bake for about 14 to 16 minutes or until the egg muffins brown around the edges and firm up. Let them cool before taking them out of the tray. Season the muffins with sea salt and black pepper and enjoy!

NUTRITION - AMOUNT PER SERVING

Calories	179	Sugar	0g
Fat	14g	Protein	12g
Carbs	1g	Cholesterol	263mg
Fiber	0g	Sodium	152mg

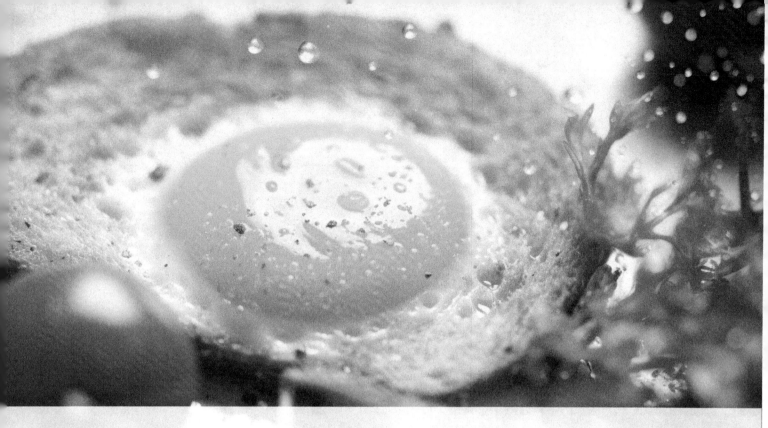

Eggs in a Hole

 10 Minutes

 2 Servings

INGREDIENTS

- 2 slices Gluten-free Bread
- 2 tsps Extra Virgin Olive Oil
- 2 Eggs (medium)

INSTRUCTIONS

1. Press a cookie cutter or the rim of a cup into the middle of your slice of bread. Remove the cutout and set it aside.

2. Heat the oil in a pan over medium heat. Toast the bread and the cutout for about 2 minutes.

3. Flip the bread and cutout, then crack the egg directly into the hole. Lower the heat, cover with a lid and cook for 4 to 5 minutes, or until your desired doneness is reached.

4. Transfer to a plate and dip the bread cutout into the egg.

NUTRITION - AMOUNT PER SERVING

Calories	189	Sugar	3g
Fat	12g	Protein	8g
Carbs	13g	Cholesterol	186mg
Fiber	1g	Sodium	199mg

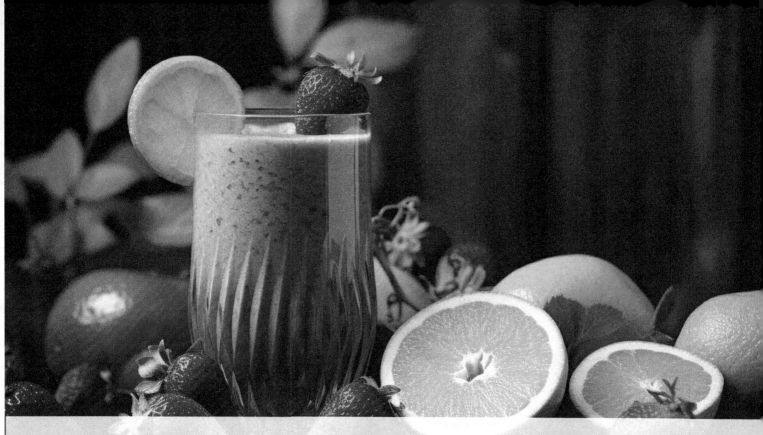

Strawberry Orange Smoothie

 5 Minutes

 1 Serving

INGREDIENTS

- 1 Navel Orange (peeled and sectioned)
- 1/2 cup Frozen Strawberries
- 1 cup Plain Coconut Milk (from the carton)

INSTRUCTIONS

1. Add all of the ingredients to a blender and blend until smooth.
2. Pour into a glass and enjoy.

NUTRITION - AMOUNT PER SERVING

Calories	186	Sugar	24g
Fat	5g	Protein	2g
Carbs	35g	Cholesterol	0mg
Fiber	5g	Sodium	40mg

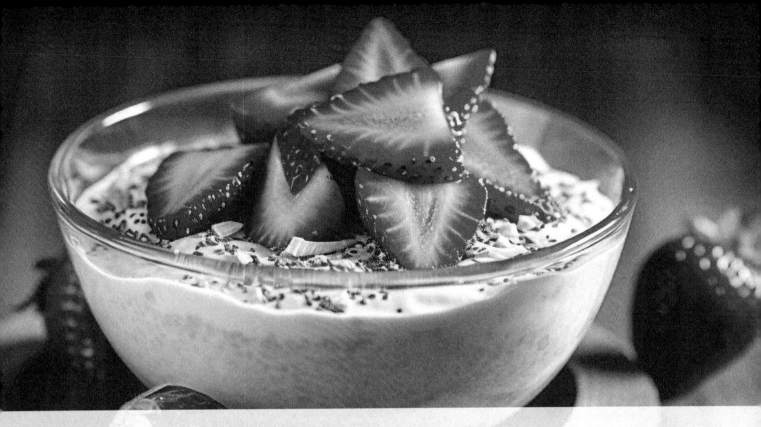

Coconut Chia Seed Yogurt

 30 Minutes

 1 Serving

INGREDIENTS

- 1 cup Unsweetened Coconut Yogurt
- 1/4 cup Chia Seeds
- 1 tsp Cinnamon
- 1/4 cup Strawberries (chopped)

INSTRUCTIONS

1. Combine the yogurt, chia seeds and cinnamon in a small bowl.
2. Mix well and refrigerate for at least 30 minutes up to overnight.
3. Top with strawberries and enjoy!

NUTRITION - AMOUNT PER SERVING

Calories	355	Sugar	3g
Fat	22g	Protein	9g
Carbs	37g	Cholesterol	0mg
Fiber	21g	Sodium	57mg

REFER TO PAGE 41 FOR THE ACCOMPANYING TOASTED WALNUTS RECIPE

Lunches

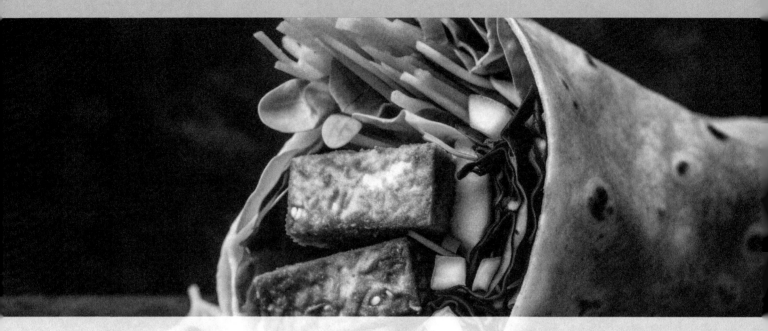

Tofu Veggie Wrap

 25 Minutes

 2 Servings

INGREDIENTS

- 282 grams Tofu (extra firm, pressed, sliced)
- 2 tbsps Tamari
- 2 Brown Rice Tortilla
- 2 cups Baby Spinach
- 1/2 Cucumber (julienned)
- 1/2 Carrot (julienned)
- 1 cup Purple Cabbage (chopped)

INSTRUCTIONS

1. Marinate the tofu slices in tamari for 15 minutes.

2. Heat a skillet or cast iron pan over medium heat. Add the drained tofu and cook for 3 to 4 minutes on each side until it becomes crispy and browned. Take it out of the pan and set it aside.

3. Place the tortilla flat and layer the spinach, cucumber, carrot, cabbage, and marinated tofu on top. Tightly roll up the wrap and enjoy!

NUTRITION - AMOUNT PER SERVING

Calories	316	Sugar	8g
Fat	10g	Protein	21g
Carbs	38g	Cholesterol	0mg
Fiber	7g	Sodium	1229mg

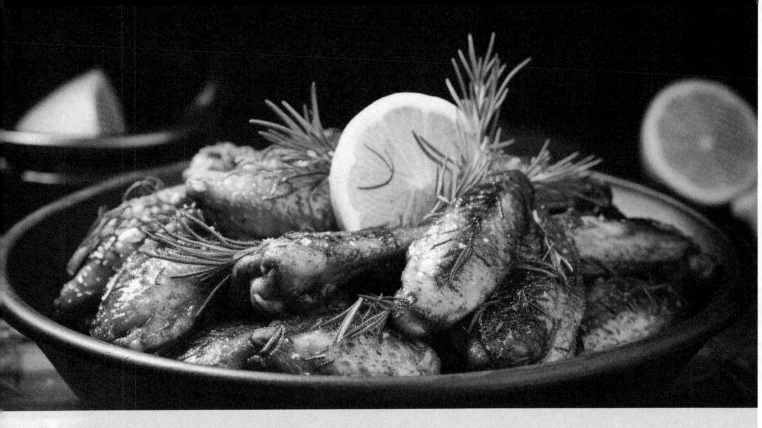

Air Fryer Lemon Dill Chicken Wings

 30 Minutes

 2 Servings

INGREDIENTS

- 1 Lemon (juiced)
- 1 tbsp Fresh Dill (chopped, plus extra for garnish)
- Sea Salt & Black Pepper (to taste)
- 340 grams Chicken Wings
- 2 grams Avocado Oil Spray

INSTRUCTIONS

1. Whisk the lemon juice, dill, salt, and pepper in a bowl. Add the chicken wings, stir, and let them marinate for at least 15 minutes.
2. Preheat the air fryer to 400°F (205°C).
3. Spray the wings with Avocado oil and place in the air fryer in a single layer. Bake for 14 to 16 minutes, flipping once, until they are crispy. Sprinkle some dill on top and enjoy!

NUTRITION - AMOUNT PER SERVING

Calories	330	Sugar	1g
Fat	22g	Protein	30g
Carbs	2g	Cholesterol	189mg
Fiber	0g	Sodium	143mg

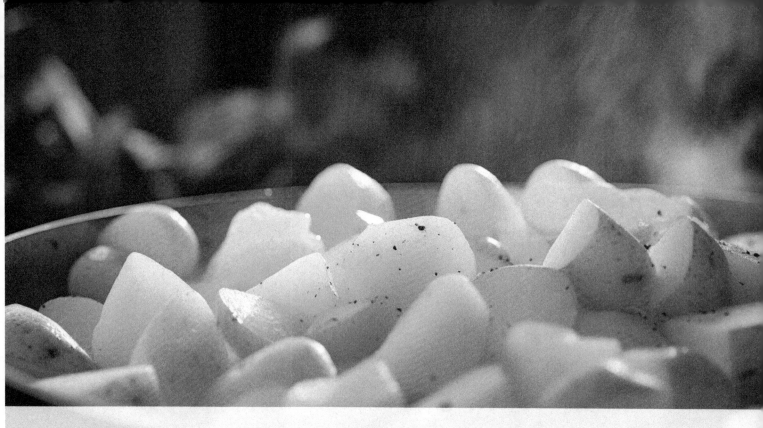

Boiled Potato

 15 minutes

 2 Servings

INGREDIENTS

- 1 Yellow Potato (medium, chopped)

INSTRUCTIONS

1. Bring a large pot of water to a boil. Add the potatoes to the pot and boil for 15 minutes or until soft.

2. Drain the water and enjoy!

NUTRITION - AMOUNT PER SERVING

Calories	82	Sugar	1g
Fat	0g	Protein	2g
Carbs	19g	Cholesterol	0mg
Fiber	2g	Sodium	6mg

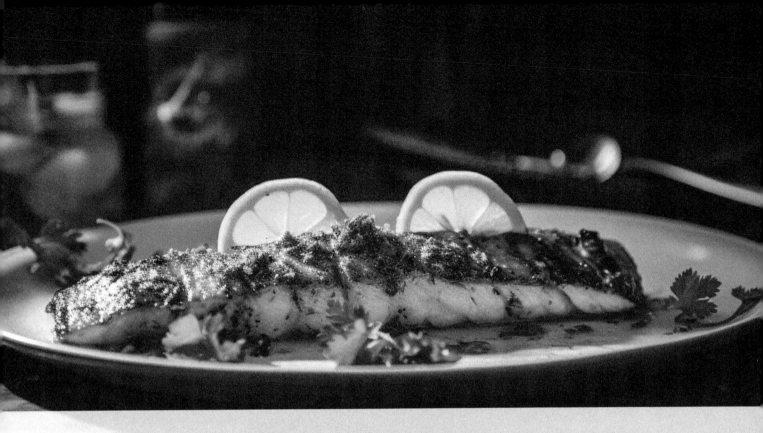

Lemon & Cilantro Baked Pickerel

 20 Minutes   **1 Serving**

INGREDIENTS

- 142 grams Pickerel Fillet
- 1 tsp Extra Virgin Olive Oil
- 1/4 Lemon (sliced)
- 1 tbsp Cilantro (coarsely chopped)
- 1/16 tsp Sea Salt

INSTRUCTIONS

1. Preheat the oven to 375°F (190°C). Line a baking sheet with parchment paper.
2. Place the pickerel fillet(s) on the baking sheet. Coat the fish in oil using a brush or your hand. Squeeze the juice from the lemon over the top of the fish, and then place the lemon slices on top. Bake for 12 to 15 minutes or until the fish is white and flakes with a fork.
3. Garnish the fish with the cilantro and salt.

NUTRITION - AMOUNT PER SERVING

Calories	167	Sugar	0g
Fat	6g	Protein	27g
Carbs	1g	Cholesterol	55mg
Fiber	0g	Sodium	203mg

REFER TO PAGE 55 FOR THE ACCOMPANYING BROWN RICE RECIPE

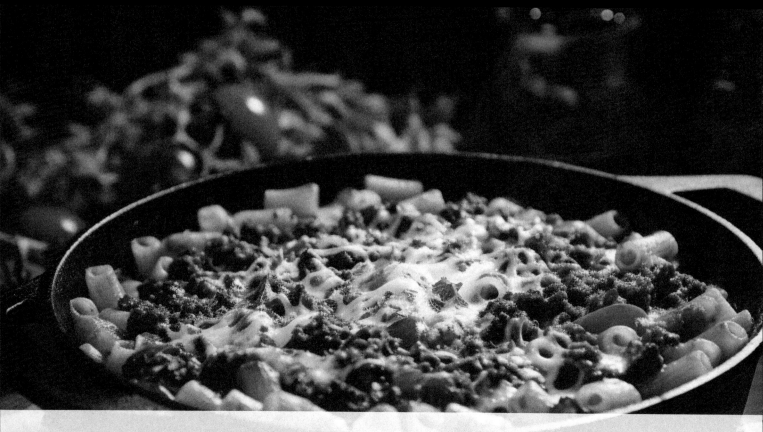

One Pot Cheeseburger Pasta

 20 Minutes

 1 Serving

INGREDIENTS

- 1/8 tsp Extra Virgin Olive Oil
- 113 grams Extra Lean Ground Beef
- 1/8 Carrot (medium, finely diced)
- 1/3 tsp Dried Basil
- 1/16 tsp Sea Salt
- 1/2 cup Diced Tomatoes (with juices)
- 1/4 cup Water
- 1/2 cup Brown Rice Macaroni (dry)
- 19 grams Cheddar Cheese (shredded)

INSTRUCTIONS

1. Heat the oil in a large pot over medium heat. Add the ground beef, diced carrot, basil, and salt. Cook for 5 minutes, stirring frequently. Drain any excess oil.

2. Stir the ingredients until they are thoroughly mixed, and the pasta is mostly under the liquid. Place a lid on top and cook for about 10 to 12 minutes, or until the pasta is completely cooked.

3. Remove the lid and stir the pasta. Top the pasta mixture with the shredded cheese and close the lid until melted.

NUTRITION - AMOUNT PER SERVING

Calories	520	Sugar	3g
Fat	20g	Protein	32g
Carbs	48g	Cholesterol	92mg
Fiber	4g	Sodium	373mg

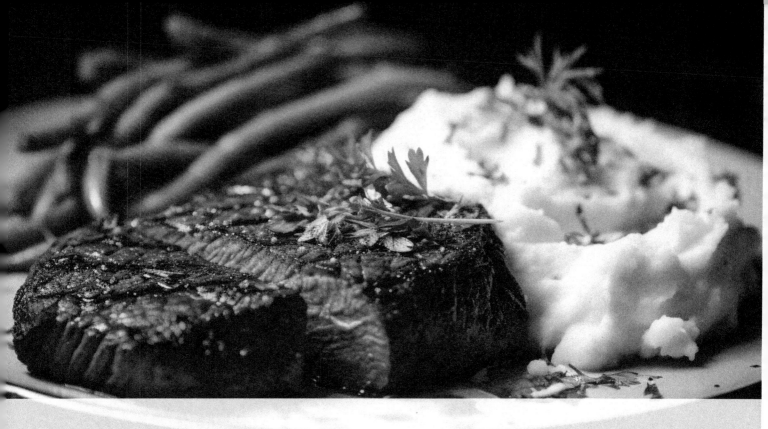

Steak, Mashed Potatoes & Green Beans

 20 Minutes

 1 Serving

INGREDIENTS

- 1 1/2 Yellow Potatoes (medium, peeled and chopped)
- 1/4 tsp Sea Salt (divided)
- 1 1/2 tsps Butter (divided)
- 113 grams Top Sirloin Steak
- 75 grams Green Beans (trimmed)
- 1 tsp Parsley (chopped)

INSTRUCTIONS

1. Add the chopped potatoes to a pot and cover with water. Boil for 10 minutes until the potatoes fall off a fork when pierced. Drain the water.
2. Add half of the salt and half of the butter to the potatoes. Mash the potatoes until they are your desired texture.
3. Season the steak with the remaining salt. Melt the rest of the butter in a cast-iron skillet on medium heat. Add the steak and cook for about 2 to 3 minutes on each side, or until the steak is cooked to your liking. Set aside and let rest for at least 5 minutes before slicing it.
4. While the steak is resting, add the green beans to the skillet and sauté for 2 to 3 minutes, or until browned.
5. Top with parsley and any remaining juices from the skillet and enjoy!

NUTRITION - AMOUNT PER SERVING

Calories	562	Sugar	5g
Fat	22g	Protein	31g
Carbs	61g	Cholesterol	103mg
Fiber	9g	Sodium	673mg

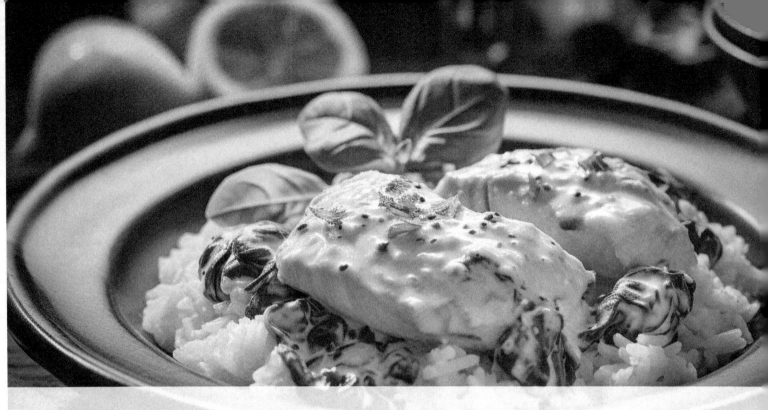

Coconut Cod & Spinach with Rice

 15 Minutes

 1 Serving

INGREDIENTS

- 1/4 cup Jasmine Rice (dry)
- 1/2 cup Canned Coconut Milk
- 1/4 cup Water
- 1 1/2 tsps Tamari
- 1 1/2 tsps Rice Vinegar
- 1 Bay Leaf
- 1/16 tsp Sea Salt (or more to taste)
- 1 Cod Fillet
- 1 cup Baby Spinach (chopped)

INSTRUCTIONS

1. Cook the rice as directed on the package and then set it aside.

2. In a saucepan combine coconut milk, water, tamari, vinegar, bay leaves, and salt over medium heat. Add the cod fillets and simmer for about 8 minutes or until the flesh is opaque.

3. Stir in spinach and remove from heat. When the spinach has wilted, serve, and enjoy.

NUTRITION - AMOUNT PER SERVING

Calories	574	Sugar	2g
Fat	23g	Protein	47g
Carbs	43g	Cholesterol	99mg
Fiber	2g	Sodium	830mg

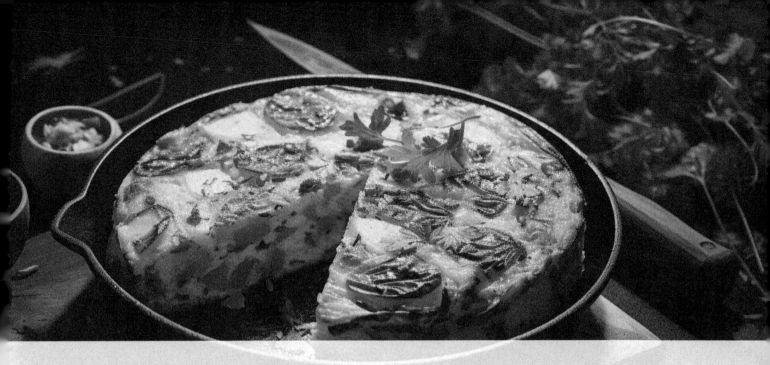

Roasted Potato Frittata

 55 Minutes

 2 Servings

INGREDIENTS

- 1 Yellow Potato (large, peeled and cut into 1/2-inch cubes)
- 2 tsps Extra Virgin Olive Oil (divided)
- 1/3 tsp Italian Seasoning
- 1/3 tsp Sea Salt (divided)
- 3 Eggs
- 1 1/3 tbsps Water

INSTRUCTIONS

1. Preheat the oven to 400°F (204°C) and line a baking sheet with parchment paper.
2. In a mixing bowl, mix the potatoes with ¾ of the oil, the Italian seasoning, and ¾ of the salt. Transfer the potato mixture onto the baking sheet and bake for approximately 30 minutes or until the potatoes turn golden brown and become tender.
3. Meanwhile, in the same mixing bowl whisk the eggs, water, and the remaining salt together. Set aside.
4. With the remaining oil, grease a cast iron skillet and heat over medium heat.
5. Move the cooked potatoes to the skillet and pour in the egg mixture. Arrange the potatoes into an even layer and let them cook for 5 minutes until the eggs start to set. Then, place the skillet in the oven and bake for 13 to 16 minutes, until the eggs are fully set.
6. Let cool slightly before slicing into equal pieces.

NUTRITION - AMOUNT PER SERVING

Calories	217	Sugar	1g
Fat	11g	Protein	11g
Carbs	19g	Cholesterol	248mg
Fiber	2g	Sodium	495mg

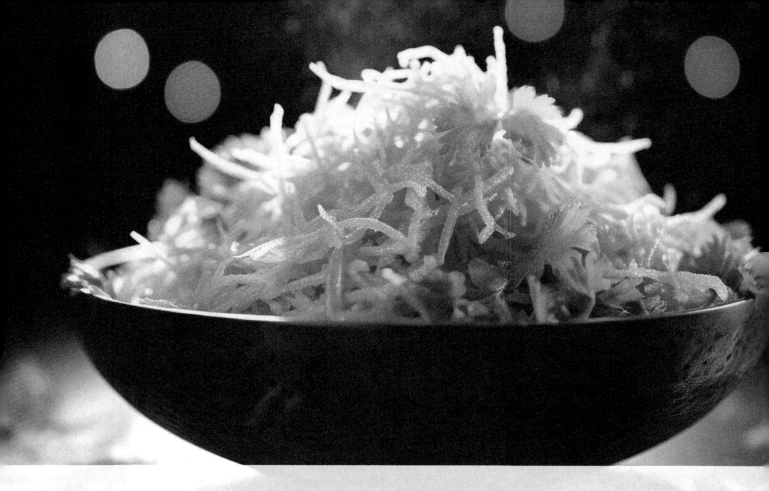

Carrot Salad

 5 Minutes

 2 Servings

INGREDIENTS

- 4 Carrots (medium, shredded)
- 2 tsps Extra Virgin Olive Oil
- 2 tsps Apple Cider Vinegar
- Sea Salt & Black Pepper (to taste)

INSTRUCTIONS

1. Add all of the ingredients to a bowl.
2. Toss to combine.

NUTRITION - AMOUNT PER SERVING

Calories	91	Sugar	6g
Fat	5g	Protein	1g
Carbs	12g	Cholesterol	0mg
Fiber	3g	Sodium	85mg

Dinners

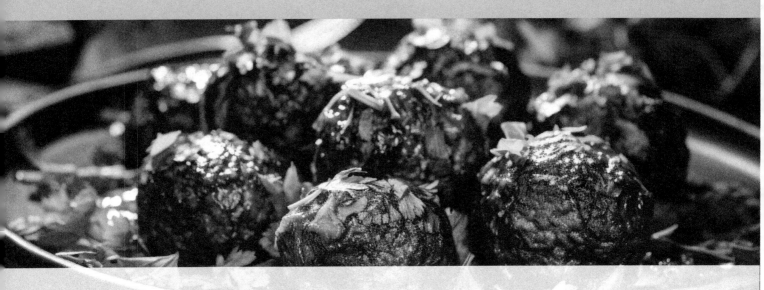

Beef Meatballs

 25 Minutes

 1 Serving

INGREDIENTS

- 226 grams Extra Lean Ground Beef
- 1/4 tsp Sea Salt
- 2 tbsps Baby Spinach (finely chopped)
- 1 tbsp Parsley (finely chopped)

INSTRUCTIONS

1. Preheat the oven to 350°F (177°C).
2. Add all ingredients into a large bowl and mix until well combined.
3. Roll into balls roughly the size of golf balls. Place in a glass baking dish, or an oven-safe dish with high sides. Bake for 20 minutes or until fully cooked.
4. Serve and enjoy!

NUTRITION - AMOUNT PER SERVING

Calories	329	Sugar	0g
Fat	16g	Protein	43g
Carbs	1g	Cholesterol	214mg
Fiber	0g	Sodium	781mg

REFER TO PAGE 55 FOR THE ACCOMPANYING BROWN RICE RECIPE

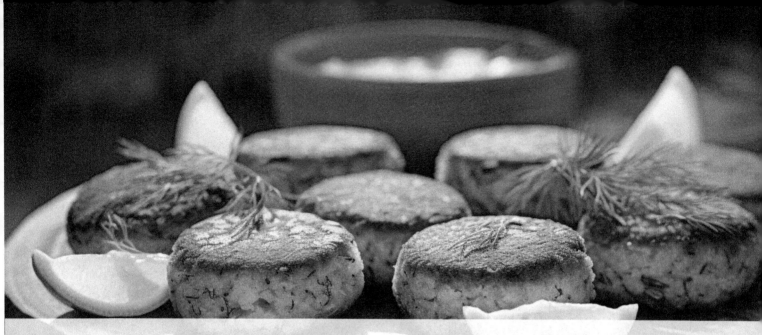

Mackerel Fish Cakes

 40 Minutes

 2 Servings

INGREDIENTS

- 2 1/3 tbsps Brown Rice (dry, rinsed)
- 1/2 cup Rice Puffs Cereal
- 1 1/3 tbsps Avocado Oil
- 76 grams Canned Mackerel
- 1 1/3 tbsps Fresh Dill (chopped)
- 1 Egg
- 1/8 tsp Sea Salt
- 1/3 Lemon (cut into wedges)

INSTRUCTIONS

1. Cook the rice according to package directions. Set aside to cool.
2. Meanwhile, in a food processor, pulse the cereal until it is a coarse crumble. Set aside in a shallow bowl.
3. Preheat a cast iron pan over medium-low heat. Add the oil 1 or 2 minutes before you are ready to cook.
4. Once the rice has cooled, add it to the food processor along with the mackerel, dill, egg, and salt. Pulse until just combined and cohesive.
5. Use a ⅓ cup measuring cup and scoop out the mixture. Gently flatten into a patty in your hands and coat in the cereal. Repeat with the remaining mixture.
6. Gently place each patty in the pan being sure not to overcrowd the pan. Adjust the heat as needed. Let the fish cakes cook for 2 or 3 minutes on each side or until a light brown crust forms. Serve with lemon wedges and enjoy!

NUTRITION - AMOUNT PER SERVING

Calories	231	Sugar	0g
Fat	14g	Protein	12g
Carbs	14g	Cholesterol	92mg
Fiber	1g	Sodium	316mg

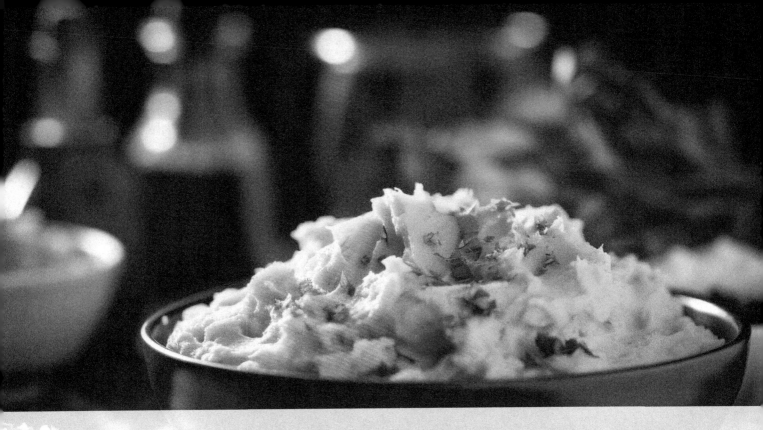

Mashed Carrots

 15 Minutes

 2 Servings

INGREDIENTS

- 6 Carrots (medium, peeled, diced)
- 2 tbsps Butter (divide)
- Sea Salt & Black Pepper (to taste)

INSTRUCTIONS

1. Add the carrots to a pot and cover with water. Bring to a boil and cook for 10 to 12 minutes or until the carrots are fork tender.
2. Drain the water and then place the carrots back into the pot. Lower the heat and add half of the butter. Mash the carrots to your desired consistency.
3. Season with salt and pepper. Transfer the mashed carrots to a serving plate. Top with remaining butter and enjoy!

NUTRITION - AMOUNT PER SERVING

Calories	177	Sugar	9g
Fat	12g	Protein	2g
Carbs	18g	Cholesterol	31mg
Fiber	5g	Sodium	128mg

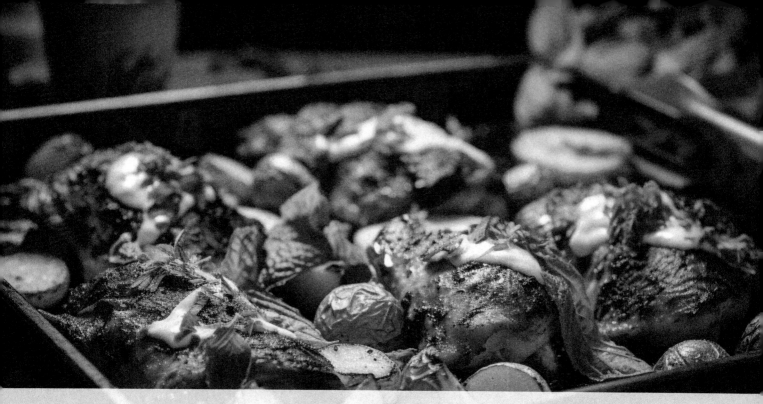

One Pan Roasted Tahini Chicken & Potato

 30 minutes

 1 Serving

INGREDIENTS

- 227 grams Chicken Thighs (boneless, skin-on)
- 1/2 Yellow Potato (large, peeled, cubed)
- 1 tsp Coconut Oil (melted)
- 1 tsp Cumin
- Sea Salt & Black Pepper
- 1 1/2 tsps Tahini
- 2 1/4 tsps Water
- 1 1/2 tsps Mint Leaves (fresh, chopped)

INSTRUCTIONS

1. Preheat the oven to 400°F (205°C). Line a baking sheet with parchment paper.
2. Place the chicken thighs and potato on the prepared baking sheet. Rub the coconut oil, cumin, salt, and pepper into the chicken and potato to coat well. Cook for 20 minutes, tossing the potato halfway through.
3. Meanwhile, mix the tahini with the water until you get a creamy consistency.
4. Drizzle the chicken and potato with the tahini sauce and garnish with mint.

NUTRITION - AMOUNT PER SERVING

Calories	450	Sugar	1g
Fat	18g	Protein	48g
Carbs	21g	Cholesterol	213mg
Fiber	3g	Sodium	235mg

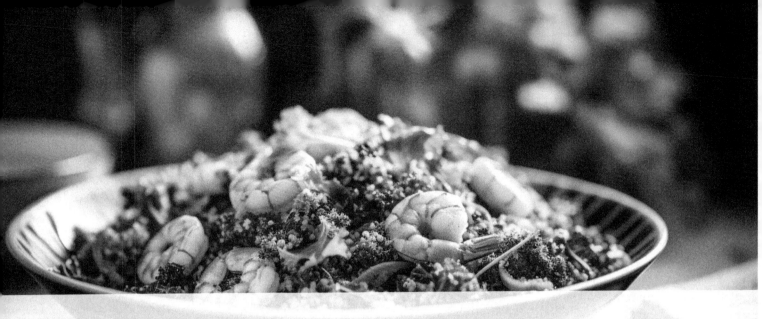

Shrimp, Kale & Quinoa Salad

 20 Minutes

 2 Servings

INGREDIENTS

- 1/4 cup Quinoa (uncooked)
- 1/2 cup Water
- Sea Salt & Black Pepper (to taste)
- 227 grams Shrimp (peeled, deveined)
- 1 tsp Cumin
- 2 tbsps Extra Virgin Olive Oil (divided)
- 1 1/2 tsps Apple Cider Vinegar
- 3/4 tsp Maple Syrup
- 1 cup Kale Leaves (stems removed and chopped)
- 1 Carrot (medium, grated or sliced)

INSTRUCTIONS

1. Boil quinoa and water in a saucepan over high heat. Reduce to a simmer and cover with a lid for 13 to 15 minutes. Season with salt and pepper, and fluff with a fork. Set aside.

2. Meanwhile, coat the shrimp with cumin, salt and pepper. Heat ¼ of the olive oil in a pan over medium-high heat. Add the shrimp and cook for about 3 to 5 minutes, flipping halfway.

3. In a large salad bowl, whisk together the vinegar, maple syrup and remaining olive oil.

4. Add the kale and carrot, and massage in the vinaigrette. Add the cooked quinoa and shrimp and toss until thoroughly combined. Divide onto plates and enjoy!

NUTRITION - AMOUNT PER SERVING

Calories	321	Sugar	3g
Fat	16g	Protein	27g
Carbs	19g	Cholesterol	183mg
Fiber	3g	Sodium	166mg

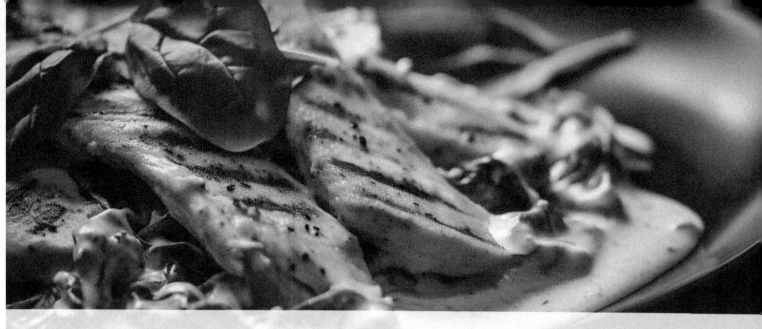

Coconut Yogurt Chicken

 2 Hours 15 Minutes

 1 Serving

INGREDIENTS

- 113 grams Chicken Breast (sliced into long strips)
- 3 tbsps Unsweetened Coconut Yogurt
- 1/2 tsp Curry Powder
- Sea Salt & Black Pepper (to taste)
- 1 1/8 tsps Extra Virgin Olive Oil
- 1 1/2 cups Baby Spinach

INSTRUCTIONS

1. Mix the chicken with the coconut yogurt, curry powder, salt, and pepper in a bowl. Put it in the fridge to marinate for at least 2 hours.

2. Add the oil to a skilled and heat over medium heat. Add the chicken strips when hot and cook for 5 to 6 minutes. Flip the strips over and cook for another 5 to 6 minutes until browned lightly.

3. Add the remaining coconut yogurt marinade to the skillet and cook for a further 2 to 3 minutes, until bubbling.

4. Toss in the spinach and stir to combine and cook until wilted, for about another 2 minutes.

5. Place the chicken and spinach onto a plate. Serve and enjoy!

NUTRITION - AMOUNT PER SERVING

Calories	215	Sugar	0g
Fat	10g	Protein	27g
Carbs	4g	Cholesterol	82mg
Fiber	2g	Sodium	96mg

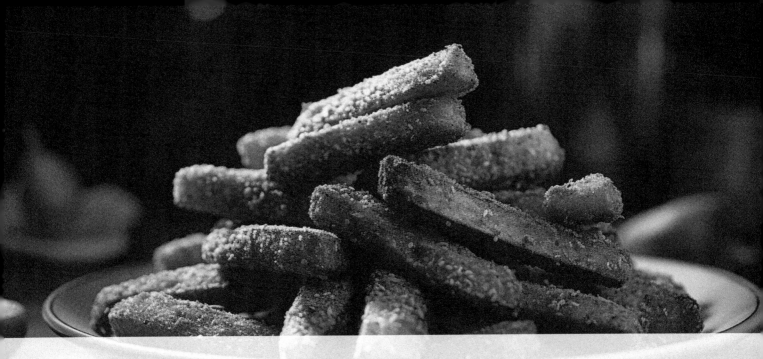

Crispy Eggplant Fries

 40 Minutes

 2 Servings

INGREDIENTS

- 1/3 Eggplant (large, cut into 1/2 inch fries)
- 2 tsps Extra Virgin Olive Oil
- 1/8 tsp Sea Salt
- 1 Egg
- 1/3 cup Cornmeal

INSTRUCTIONS

1. Preheat the oven to 425°F (220°C) and line a baking sheet with parchment paper.

2. Add the eggplant fries to a mixing bowl and toss with the oil and salt until well coated.

3. Whisk the egg in a small or shallow bowl. Place the cornmeal on a plate or in a second shallow bowl.

4. A few fries at a time, dip the eggplant in the egg, and shake off any excess. Then dip the egg-coated eggplant in the cornmeal to evenly coat all sides. Shake off any excess cornmeal and place the fries on the prepared baking sheet. Repeat until all the eggplant is used up. Discard any excess egg or cornmeal.

5. Bake for 22 to 25 minutes, flipping halfway through, or until the fries are golden brown and very crispy. Season with additional salt if needed and enjoy!

NUTRITION - AMOUNT PER SERVING

Calories	160	Sugar	3g
Fat	7g	Protein	5g
Carbs	21g	Cholesterol	62mg
Fiber	4g	Sodium	229mg

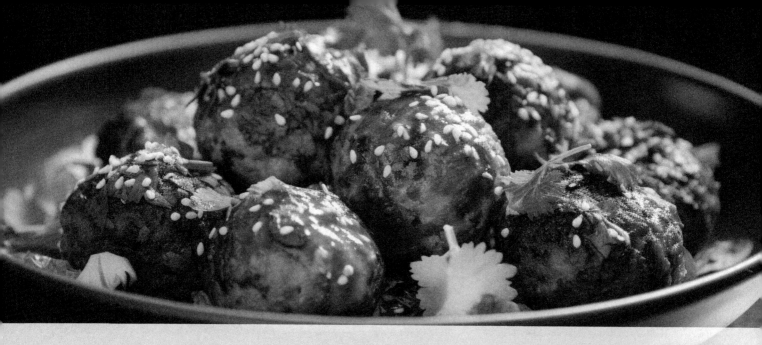

Chicken & Quinoa Meatballs

 35 Minutes

 2 Servings

INGREDIENTS

- 2 tbsps Quinoa (uncooked)
- 1/4 cup Water
- 1/2 Egg
- 227 grams Extra Lean Ground Chicken
- 1/4 cup Cilantro (chopped)
- 1/2 tsp Ginger (fresh, minced)
- 1 tsp Fish Sauce
- 1/2 tsp Coconut Sugar
- 1/4 Lime (juice and zest)
- 1 tbsp Brown Rice Flour

INSTRUCTIONS

1. Place the quinoa and water in a saucepan over medium-high heat and bring to a boil. Once boiling, cover and reduce heat to low. Let it simmer for 12 minutes. Remove from heat, fluff with a fork and set aside.

2. Preheat the oven to 400°F (204°C) and line a baking sheet with parchment paper.

3. In a large bowl, add the egg and beat with a fork. To the same bowl, add the chicken, cilantro, ginger, fish sauce, coconut sugar, lime juice and zest and mix well. Add the quinoa and the rice flour and mix again.

4. Roll the chicken mixture into balls slightly bigger than a golf ball. Place them on the baking sheet and bake for 18 to 20 minutes. Remove, serve and enjoy!

NUTRITION - AMOUNT PER SERVING

Calories	243	Sugar	1g
Fat	11g	Protein	23g
Carbs	12g	Cholesterol	144mg
Fiber	1g	Sodium	324mg

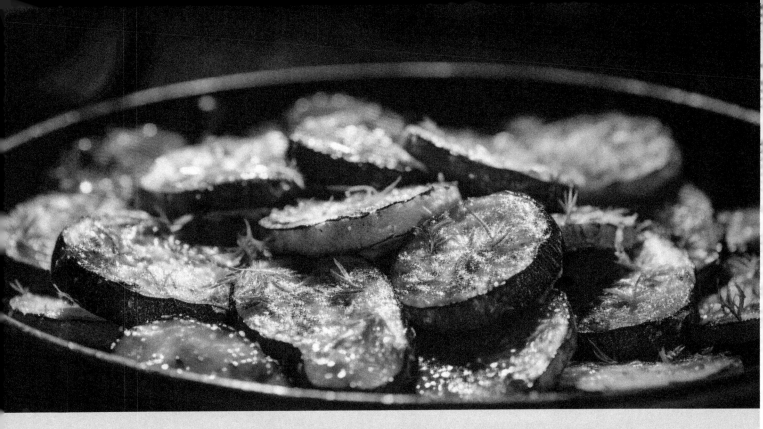

Pan Fried Zucchini

 10 Minutes

 2 Servings

INGREDIENTS

- 1 tbsp Coconut Oil
- 75 grams Zucchini (medium, sliced into rounds)
- ¼ tsp Sea Salt (or more to taste)

INSTRUCTIONS

1. Heat oil in a skillet over medium-high heat.
2. Add the zucchini slices and cook for about 3-5 minutes each side, or until brown.
3. Season with salt and enjoy!

NUTRITION - AMOUNT PER SERVING

Calories	69	Sugar	1g
Fat	7g	Protein	0g
Carbs	2g	Cholesterol	0mg
Fiber	0g	Sodium	295mg

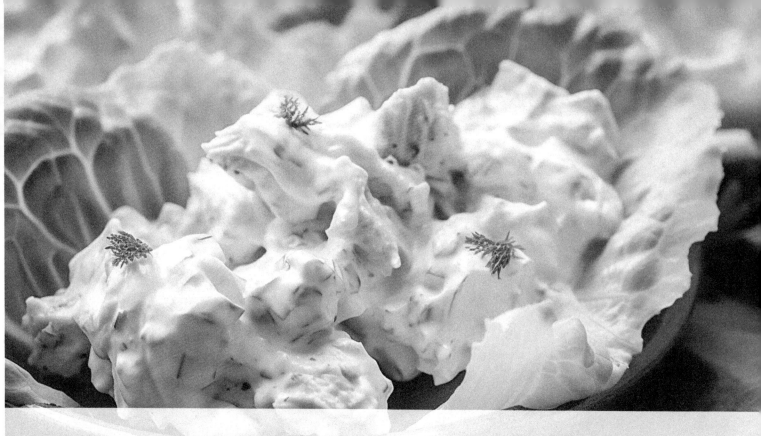

Creamy Herb Chicken Lettuce Wraps

 10 Minutes

 2 Servings

INGREDIENTS

- 227 grams Chicken Breast, Cooked (chopped)
- 1/2 cup Unsweetened Coconut Yogurt
- 2 tbsps Fresh Dill (finely chopped)
- 2 tbsps Parsley (finely chopped)
- 1/2 tsp Sea Salt (to taste)
- 1/8 head Green Lettuce (leaves separated)

INSTRUCTIONS

1. In a bowl, combine the chicken, coconut yogurt, dill, parsley, and salt.

2. Fill the lettuce leaves with creamy herb chicken and enjoy!

NUTRITION - AMOUNT PER SERVING

Calories	201	Sugar	0g
Fat	5g	Protein	35g
Carbs	3g	Cholesterol	118mg
Fiber	1g	Sodium	664mg

Snacks

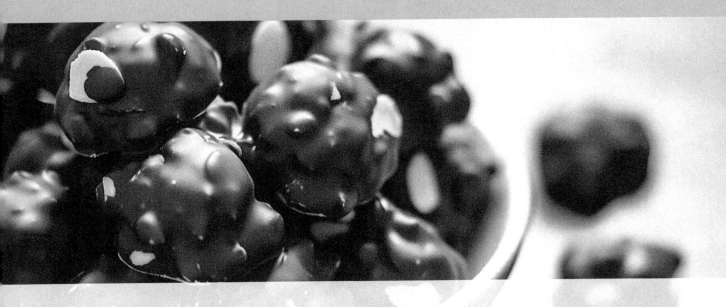

Macadamia Nut Clusters

 30 Minutes

 3 Servings

INGREDIENTS

- 60 grams Dark Chocolate (chopped)
- 4 ½ tbsps Macadamia Nuts
- ¼ tsp Sea Salt (coarse)

INSTRUCTIONS

1. Add the dark chocolate to a microwave-safe bowl. Microwave for one minute, then stir. Continue to microwave for 30-second increments, stirring after each 30-second period, until all the chocolate has melted.
2. Cover a baking sheet with parchment paper. Arrange the macadamia nuts into groups of five or six nuts. Scoop the melted chocolate over the top until each macadamia cluster is covered. Sprinkle with sea salt to taste.
3. Refrigerate for at least 20 minutes or until the chocolate has hardened.

NUTRITION - AMOUNT PER SERVING

Calories	206	Sugar	5g
Fat	18g	Protein	3g
Carbs	11g	Cholesterol	1mg
Fiber	3g	Sodium	78mg

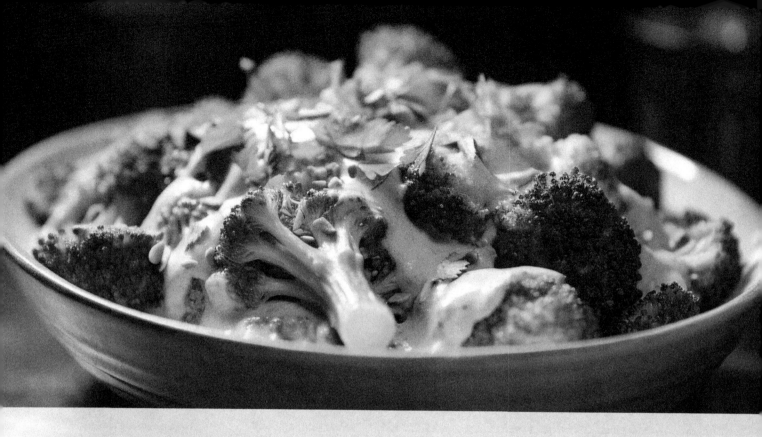

Creamy Spiced Broccoli

 10 Minutes

 1 Serving

INGREDIENTS

- 65 grams Broccoli Florets (small)
- 1/3 cup Unsweetened Coconut Yogurt
- 3/4 tsp Curry Powder
- Sea Salt & Black Pepper (to taste)

INSTRUCTIONS

1. Add the broccoli to a steamer basket over boiling water. Steam for 4 to 5 minutes or until the broccoli is tender.

2. Meanwhile, in a bowl combine the coconut yogurt and curry powder. Season with salt and pepper to taste.

3. Add the steamed broccoli to the bowl with the spiced coconut yogurt and mix to evenly coat the broccoli. Serve and enjoy!

NUTRITION - AMOUNT PER SERVING

Calories	21	Sugar	0g
Fat	1g	Protein	1g
Carbs	3g	Cholesterol	0mg
Fiber	1g	Sodium	13mg

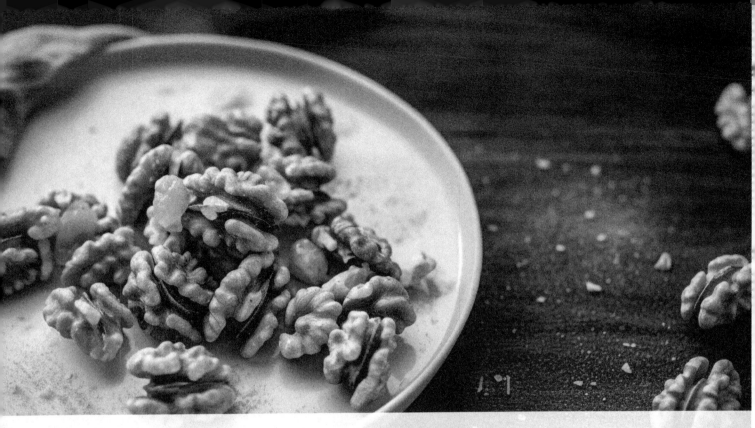

Cheezy Walnuts

 5 Minutes

 1 Serving

INGREDIENTS

- ¼ cup Walnuts
- 1 ½ tsps Avocado Oil
- ½ tsp Nutritional Yeast
- ⅛ tsp Sea Salt

INSTRUCTIONS

1. In a bowl, toss the walnuts with the oil until well coated.

2. Sprinkle the nutritional yeast and sea salt over the top and enjoy!

NUTRITION - AMOUNT PER SERVING

Calories	264	Sugar	1g
Fat	27g	Protein	5g
Carbs	5g	Cholesterol	0mg
Fiber	2g	Sodium	300mg

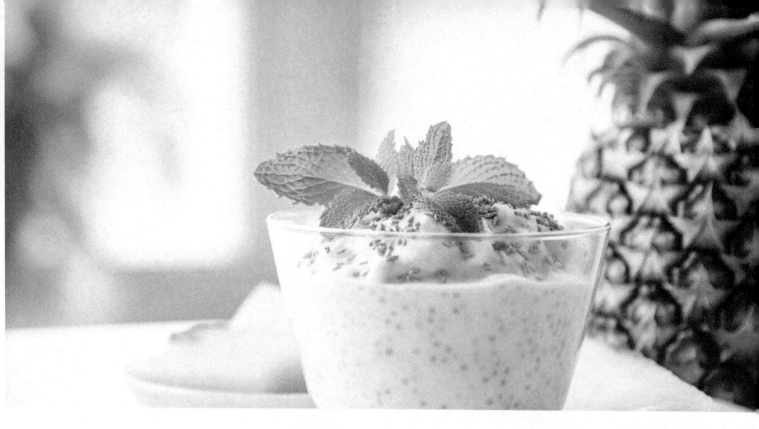

Pineapple Chia Pudding

 35 Minutes

 1 Serving

INGREDIENTS

- 1/4 cup Canned Coconut Milk
- 59 milliliters Pineapple Juice
- 2 tbsps Chia Seeds
- 1/4 Lime (zested)
- 2 2/3 tbsps Pineapple (chopped)
- 1 1/2 tsps Mint Leaves (chopped, optional garnish)

INSTRUCTIONS

1. Combine the coconut milk, pineapple juice, chia seeds, and lime zest in a bowl.

2. Refrigerate for at least 30 minutes or until chilled and the chia seeds have set.

3. Stir well, then serve in a glass. Top with pineapple and mint, if using.

NUTRITION - AMOUNT PER SERVING

Calories	260	Sugar	9g
Fat	18g	Protein	5g
Carbs	22g	Cholesterol	0mg
Fiber	8g	Sodium	20mg

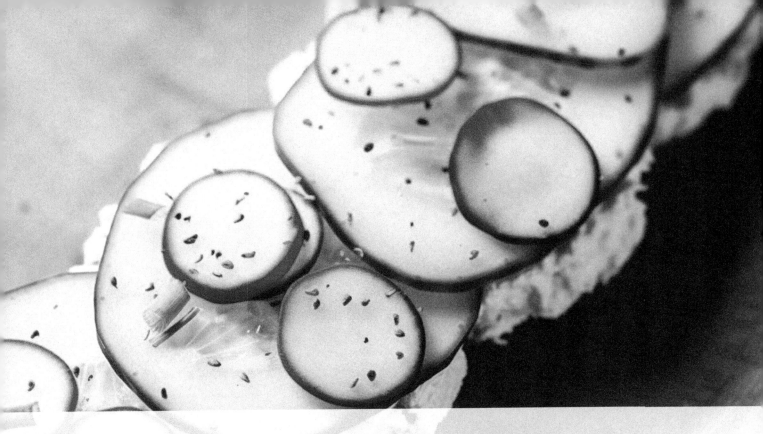

Radish & Cucumber Rice Cakes

 10 Minutes

 2 Servings

INGREDIENTS

- 4 Brown Rice Cakes
- ½ cup Radishes (sliced)
- ½ Cucumber (sliced)
- Sea Salt & Black Pepper (to taste)

INSTRUCTIONS

1. Top each rice cake with radishes and cucumber.
2. Sprinkle with salt and pepper and enjoy!

NUTRITION - AMOUNT PER SERVING

Calories	136	Sugar	2g
Fat	1g	Protein	3g
Carbs	32g	Cholesterol	0mg
Fiber	3g	Sodium	13mg

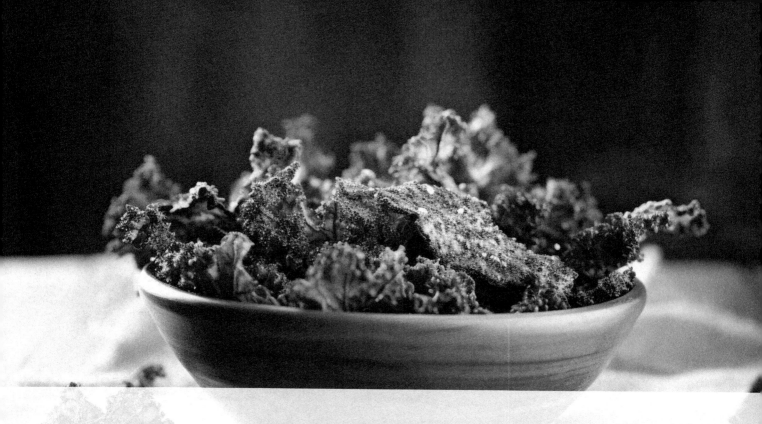

Sea Salted Coconut Kale Chips

 20 Minutes

 4 Servings

INGREDIENTS

- 1 cup Kale Leaves
- 1 tbsp Coconut Oil (melted)
- 1 tsp Sea Salt
- 1/2 Lemon (juiced)

INSTRUCTIONS

1. Preheat oven to 350°F (177°C). Use a sharp knife to cut your kale leaves into large pieces. They shrink up in the oven, so don't cut them too small!

2. Place kale in a large bowl. Drizzle with lemon juice and melted coconut oil. Season with desired amount of sea salt. Use clean hands to massage all ingredients into kale.

3. Line a large baking sheet with parchment paper. Place the kale leaves in a single layer. Don't overcrowd. You will have to bake in batches for the perfect chips.

4. Cook in oven for 10 to 15 minutes. Remove from oven when crisp.

NUTRITION - AMOUNT PER SERVING

Calories	33	Sugar	0g
Fat	3g	Protein	0g
Carbs	1g	Cholesterol	0mg
Fiber	0g	Sodium	593mg

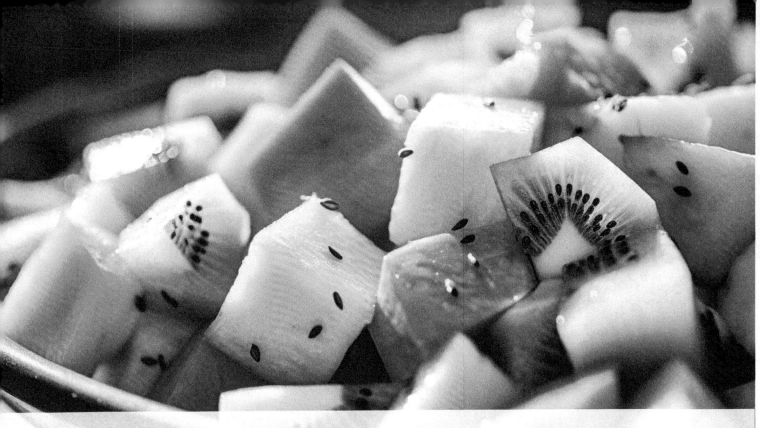

Tropical Fruit Salad

 5 Minutes

 2 Servings

INGREDIENTS

- 1 cup Papaya
- 1 Kiwi (peeled, chopped)
- 1 cup Pineapple
- 2 tsps Maple Syrup
- 1/2 tsp Cinnamon
- 1/4 tsp Cardamom

INSTRUCTIONS

1. Add the papaya, kiwi, pineapple, and maple syrup to a bowl. Toss to combine.

2. Sprinkle the cinnamon and cardamom on top and mix again.

3. Divide into bowls and enjoy!

NUTRITION - AMOUNT PER SERVING

Calories	112	Sugar	21g
Fat	0g	Protein	1g
Carbs	29g	Cholesterol	0mg
Fiber	4g	Sodium	8mg

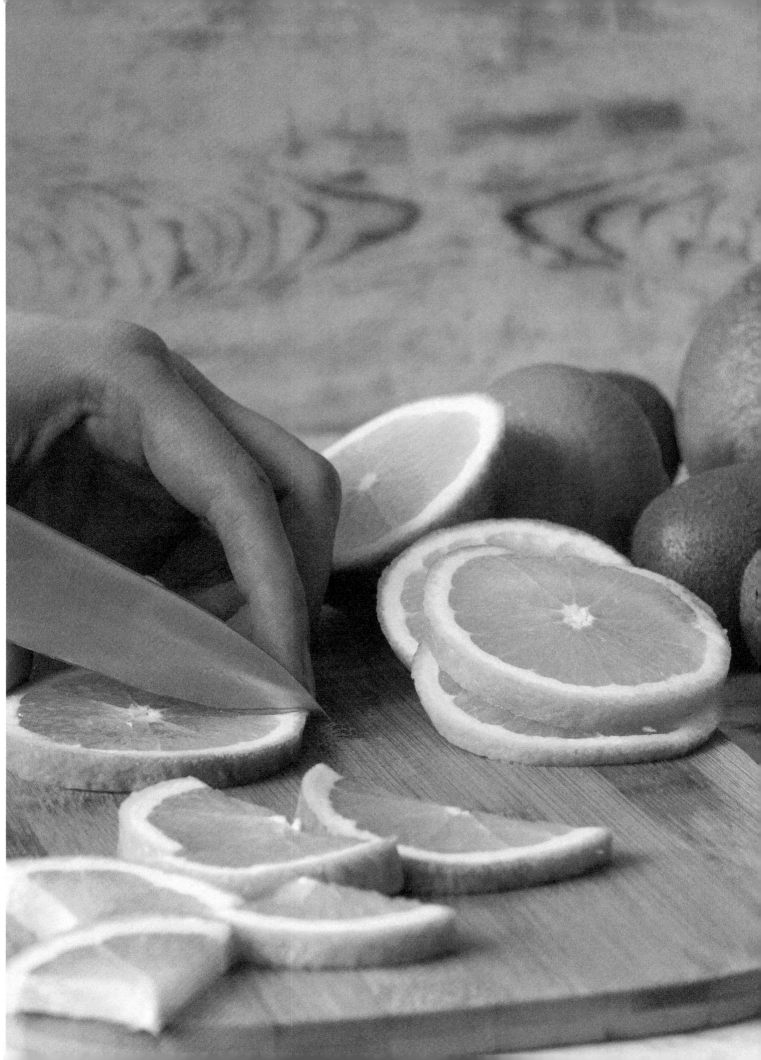

WEEK 3

7-Days Meal Plan

MONDAY

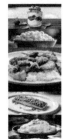

BREAKFAST
Coconut Yogurt Parfait, Macadamia Nuts

LUNCH
Sweet & Sour Chicken with Broccoli

DINNER
Walnut Crusted Salmon, Mashed Potatoes

SNACKS
Pineapple with Cinnamon

TUESDAY

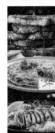

BREAKFAST
Sweet & Savory French Toast

LUNCH
Carrot & Parsley Omelet

DINNER
Maple Dijon Chicken & Lemon Herb Rice

SNACKS
Sea Salt Spinach Chips

WEDNESDAY

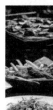

BREAKFAST
Sheet Pan Strawberry Pancakes

LUNCH
Chicken Fingers & Fries

DINNER
Lemony Shrimp Pasta

SNACKS
Radishes & Swiss Cheese

THURSDAY

BREAKFAST
Pineapple Yogurt Bowl, Pumpkin Seeds Spoons

LUNCH
Strawberry Kiwi Salad with Chicken

DINNER
Marinated Eggplant with Quinoa

SNACKS
Sesame Cucumber Salad

FRIDAY

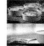

BREAKFAST
Air Fryer Broccoli & Cheddar Quiche Cups, Coconut Matcha Latte

LUNCH
Greek Pasta Salad

DINNER
Chicken & Potato Casserole

SNACKS
Dark Chocolate Peanut Butter Cups

SATURDAY

BREAKFAST
Flourless Peanut Butter Pancakes, Golden Smoothie

LUNCH
Tofu Veggie Fried Rice

DINNER
Broiled Lemon & Pepper Sole, Quinoa

SNACKS
Orange Popsicles

SUNDAY

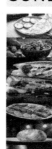

BREAKFAST
Plain Omelet with Cucumber, Toasted Walnuts

LUNCH
Broccoli, Chicken & Cheese Melt

DINNER
Slow Roasted Salmon with Citrus, Baked Potato

SNACKS
Kiwi, Yogurt & Maple Syrup

Shopping List

FRUITS
3 Kiwi
¾ Lemon
2 ⅔ tbsps Lemon Juice
¼ Navel Orange
1 cup Papaya
3 cups Pineapple
½ cup Strawberries
125 grams Strawberries

SEEDS, NUTS & SPICES
¼ tsp Chili Powder
1 ⅔ tsps Cinnamon
⅔ tsp Dried Basil
½ tsp Italian Seasoning
⅓ cupMacadamia Nuts
¾ tsp Oregano
¼ tsp Paprika
2 tbsps Pumpkin Seeds
Sea Salt & Black Pepper
1 tsp Sesame Seeds
2 tbsps Sunflower Seeds
2 tsps Turmeric
1 cup Walnuts

FROZEN
2 cups Frozen Broccoli
2 cups Frozen Pineapple

VEGETABLES
1 cup Arugula
3 cups Baby Spinach
1 ⅔ cups Broccoli
1 ¼ Carrots
¾ cup Cherry Tomatoes
3 tbsps Cilantro
1 ¾ Cucumber
75 grams Eggplant
⅛ bulb Fennel
1 tbsp Ginger
1 cup Grated Carrot
1 ⅓ tbsps Parsley

¼ cup Purple Cabbage
1 cup Radishes
3 ⅓ Russet Potato
1/16 tsp Thyme
½ Yellow Potato
1 ⅛ Zucchini

PANTRY STAPLES
¾ cup Beef Broth
¾ cup Brown Rice Pasta
    Shells
¼ cup Brown Rice Spaghetti
½ cup Crushed Pineapple
1 ¾ cups Jasmine Rice
1 ¼ cups Quinoa
2 tsps Tomato Paste
⅓ cup All Natural Peanut
    Butter
1 tsp Green Tea Powder
¾ cup Maple Syrup

BAKING
1 tsp Arrowroot Powder
1 ½ tsps Baking Powder
⅔ cup Brown Rice Flour
15 grams Dark Chocolate
1 tbsp Unsweetened
    Shredded Coconut
½ tsp Vanilla Extract

BREAD, FISH, MEAT & CHEESE
163 grams Cheddar Cheese
874 grams Chicken Breast
160 grams Chicken Breast,
    Cooked
136 grams Extra Lean
    Ground Beef
113 grams Extra Lean Ground
    Chicken
4 slices Gluten-free Bread
340 grams Salmon Fillet

114 grams Shrimp
227 grams Sole Fillet
99 grams Sourdough Bread
45 grams Swiss Cheese
114 grams Tofu

CONDIMENTS & OILS
3 ⅔ tbsps Apple Cider
    Vinegar
1 tbsp Avocado Oil
1 gram Avocado Oil Spray
1 tbsp Coconut Aminos
1 tbsp Coconut Butter
1 tbsp Coconut Oil
1 tbsp Dijon Mustard
½ cup Extra Virgin Olive Oil
2 ⅔ tbsps Pitted Kalamata
    Olives
2 ¼ tsps Red Wine Vinegar
2 ¾ tbsps Rice Vinegar
1 ⅛ tsps Sesame Oil
2 ½ tbsps Tamari

FRIDGE
1 ¾ tbsps Butter
15 Eggs
1 ½ cups Orange Juice
½ cup Plain Coconut Milk
3 ½ cups Unsweetened
    Almond Milk
2 ½ cups Unsweetened
    Coconut Yogurt

Breakfasts

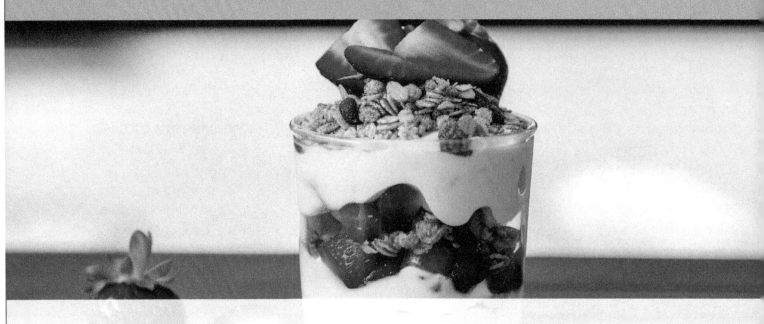

Coconut Yogurt Parfait

 5 Minutes

 1 Serving

INGREDIENTS

- 1 cup Unsweetened Coconut Yogurt (divided)
- 2 tbsps Walnuts (roughly chopped, divided)
- 1/2 cup Strawberries (chopped, divided)

INSTRUCTIONS

1. Place half the coconut yogurt in a glass jar or bowl.

2. Top with half the walnuts and half the strawberries. Add the remaining coconut yogurt, walnuts and strawberries.

3. Serve and enjoy!

NUTRITION - AMOUNT PER SERVING

Calories	231	Sugar	5g
Fat	17g	Protein	4g
Carbs	20g	Cholesterol	0mg
Fiber	5g	Sodium	51mg

REFER TO PAGE 45 FOR THE ACCOMPANYING MACADAMIA NUTS RECIPE

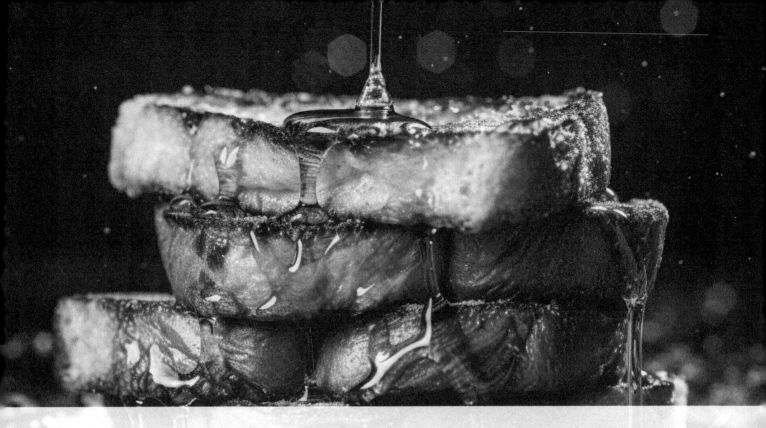

Sweet & Savory French Toast

 15 Minutes

 2 Servings

INGREDIENTS

- 2 Eggs
- 1/4 cup Unsweetened Almond Milk
- 1 tbsp Coconut Aminos
- 4 slices Gluten-free Bread
- 1 tbsp Extra Virgin Olive Oil
- 2 tbsps Maple Syrup

INSTRUCTIONS

1. Whisk together the eggs, milk, and coconut aminos in a bowl. Dip the bread slices into the egg mixture, coating both sides evenly.

2. Heat the oil on a nonstick griddle or skillet over medium heat. Cook the bread slices for about 3 to 5 minutes per side, or until browned. Repeat the process until all the bread is cooked.

3. Divide onto plates and top with maple syrup.

NUTRITION - AMOUNT PER SERVING

Calories	349	Sugar	119g
Fat	17g	Protein	10g
Carbs	40g	Cholesterol	186mg
Fiber	3g	Sodium	484mg

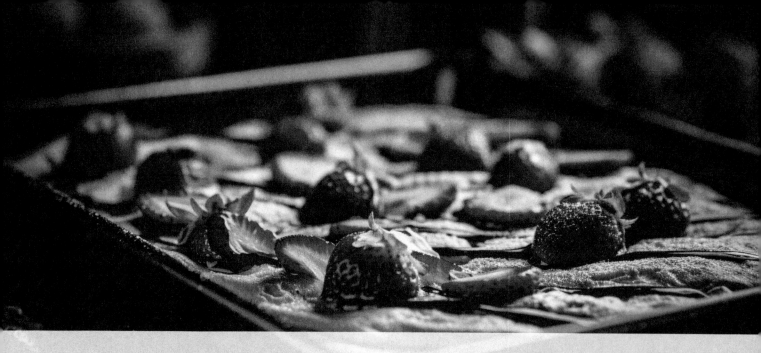

Sheet Pan Strawberry Pancakes

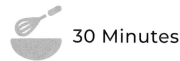 30 Minutes

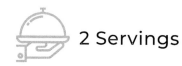 2 Servings

INGREDIENTS

- 1/2 cup Unsweetened Almond Milk
- 1 1/2 tsps Apple Cider Vinegar
- 2 Eggs
- 2 tsps Maple Syrup
- 1/2 tsp Vanilla Extract
- 2/3 cupBrown Rice Flour
- 1 tsp Baking Powder
- 2/3 tsp Cinnamon
- 2 tsps Coconut Oil (melted)
- 65 grams Strawberries (sliced, fresh or frozen)

INSTRUCTIONS

1. Preheat the oven to 425°F (220°C) and line a large baking sheet with parchment paper.

2. Mix the almond milk and apple cider vinegar in a bowl, stirring well. Let the milk sit for approximately 5 minutes to sour.

3. Whisk in the eggs, maple syrup, and vanilla extract into the soured milk until combined.

4. Whisk in the flour, baking powder, and cinnamon, and when almost combined stir in the coconut oil and continue stirring until the batter is smooth.

5. Transfer the batter to the baking sheet and spread it into an even layer. Top the batter with the strawberry slices. Bake for 13 to 15 minutes or until the pancake is spongy to the touch or when an inserted knife or toothpick comes out clean.

6. Allow the pancake to cool slightly then cut into squares and enjoy!

NUTRITION - AMOUNT PER SERVING

Calories	321	Sugar	6g
Fat	10g	Protein	9g
Carbs	49g	Cholesterol	124mg
Fiber	4g	Sodium	337mg

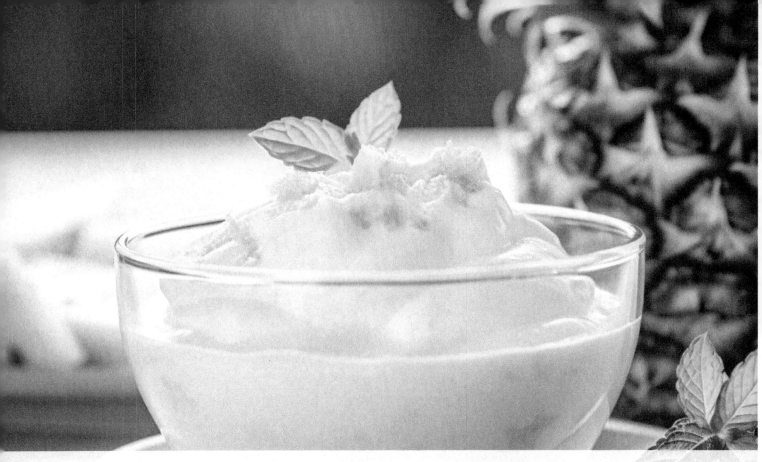

Pineapple Yogurt Bowl

 5 Minutes

 2 Servings

INGREDIENTS

- 1 cup Unsweetened Coconut Yogurt
- 1 cup Pineapple (chopped)
- 1 tbsp Unsweetened Shredded Coconut (optional)

INSTRUCTIONS

1. Divide the coconut yogurt between bowls and top with the pineapple and shredded coconut (if using).

NUTRITION - AMOUNT PER SERVING

Calories	113	Sugar	9g
Fat	5g	Protein	1g
Carbs	17g	Cholesterol	0mg
Fiber	3g	Sodium	26mg

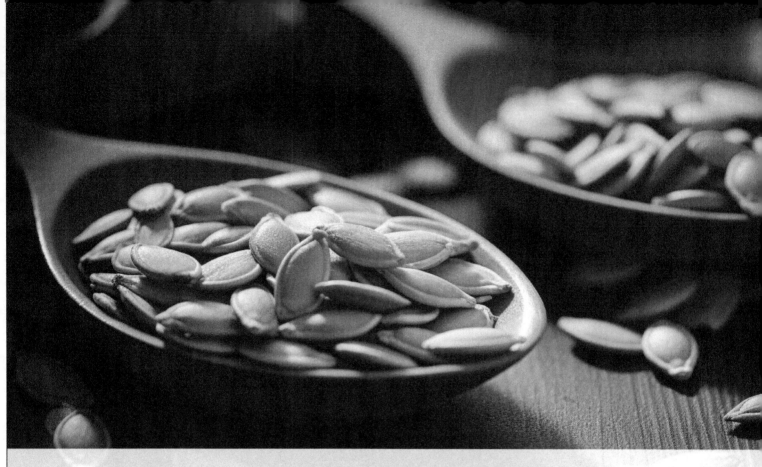

Pumpkin Seeds Spoons

 1 Minute

 1 Serving

INGREDIENTS

- 2 tbsps Pumpkin Seeds

INSTRUCTIONS

1. Place in a bowl and enjoy!

NUTRITION - AMOUNT PER SERVING

Calories	90	Sugar	0g
Fat	8g	Protein	5g
Carbs	2g	Cholesterol	0mg
Fiber	1g	Sodium	1mg

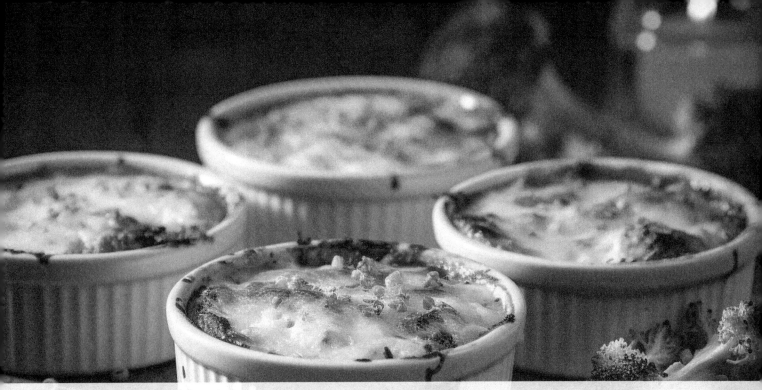

Air Fryer Broccoli & Cheddar Quiche Cups

 20 Minutes

 2 Servings

INGREDIENTS

- 1 gram Avocado Oil Spray
- 4 Eggs (whisked)
- Sea Salt & Black Pepper (to taste)
- ⅔ cup Broccoli (florets, chopped very small)
- 47 grams Cheddar Cheese (grated, divided)

INSTRUCTIONS

1. Preheat the air fryer to 300°F (150°C) and grease ramekin(s) with oil spray.
2. Season the whisked eggs with salt and pepper. Add the broccoli and ¾ of the cheese to the eggs and mix to combine.
3. Divide the egg mixture evenly between the ramekin(s) and place in the air fryer. Bake for 13 to 14 minutes, until cooked through.
4. Top with the remaining cheese and increase the temperature to 380°F (195°C). Bake for 2 minutes longer or until the cheese has melted.
5. Carefully remove from the air fryer.

NUTRITION - AMOUNT PER SERVING

Calories	249	Sugar	1g
Fat	18g	Protein	19g
Carbs	4g	Cholesterol	395mg
Fiber	1g	Sodium	307mg

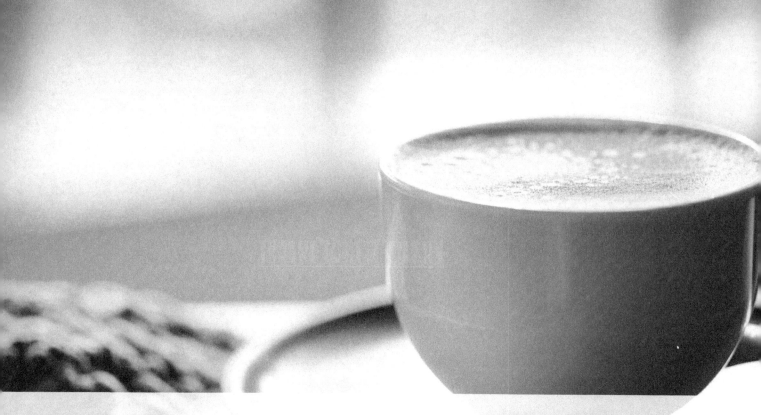

Coconut Matcha Latte

 10 Minutes

 1 Serving

INGREDIENTS

- 1 cup Water (hot)
- 1/2 cup Plain Coconut Milk
- 1 tsp Green Tea Powder
- 1 tbsp Coconut Butter
- 1 tbsp Maple Syrup

INSTRUCTIONS

1. Add the hot water, coconut milk, matcha, coconut butter, and maple syrup to a blender.
2. Blend until creamy and frothy. Pour into a mug and enjoy!

NUTRITION - AMOUNT PER SERVING

Calories	197	Sugar	17g
Fat	13g	Protein	1g
Carbs	21g	Cholesterol	0mg
Fiber	2g	Sodium	30mg

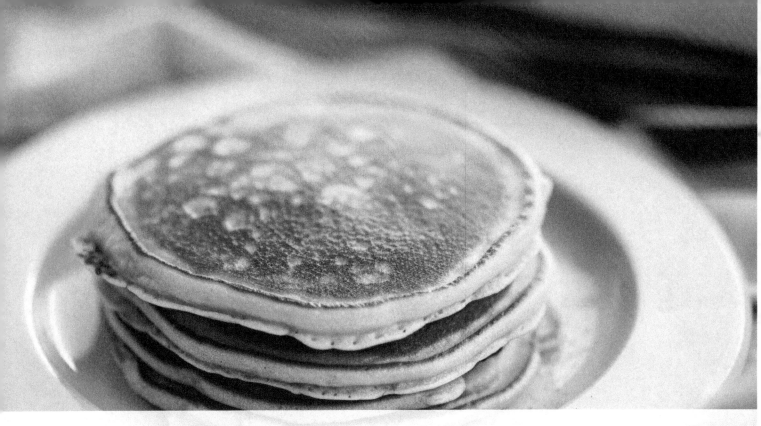

Flourless Peanut Butter Pancakes

 15 Minutes

 2 Servings

INGREDIENTS

- ¼ cup All Natural Peanut Butter
- 2 tbsps Unsweetened Almond Milk
- 1 Egg
- ½ tsp Baking Powder
- ½ tsp Coconut Oil (for the pan)

INSTRUCTIONS

1. Add the peanut butter, milk, and egg to a bowl and whisk together until a smooth batter forms. Then, stir in the baking powder.

2. Heat a pan over medium heat. Add the coconut oil once the pan is hot. Use a spoon to ladle the batter into the pan, making small ¼ cup portions to create small pancakes. Cook the pancakes for approximately 3 to 5 minutes on each side or until they turn golden brown and are fully cooked.

3. Continue using the remaining batter, adding more oil to the pan as necessary.

4. Divide pancakes between plates and enjoy!

NUTRITION - AMOUNT PER SERVING

Calories	241	Sugar	3g
Fat	20g	Protein	10g
Carbs	8g	Cholesterol	93mg
Fiber	2g	Sodium	173mg

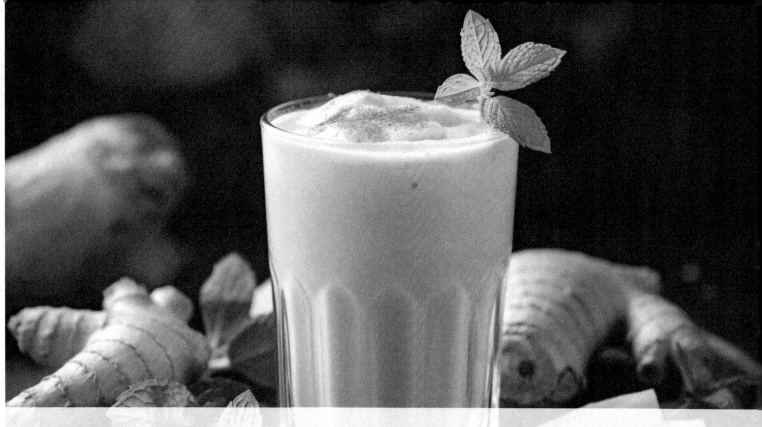

Golden Smoothie

 5 Minutes

 2 Servings

INGREDIENTS

- 2 cups Unsweetened Almond Milk
- 2 cups Frozen Pineapple
- 1 cup Papaya
- 1 Zucchini (chopped and peeled)
- 1 tbsp Ginger (fresh, minced)
- 2 tsps Turmeric

INSTRUCTIONS

1. Place all ingredients in your blender and blend until smooth.
2. Pour into a glass and enjoy!

NUTRITION - AMOUNT PER SERVING

Calories	170	Sugar	24g
Fat	3g	Protein	4g
Carbs	36g	Cholesterol	0mg
Fiber	6g	Sodium	177mg

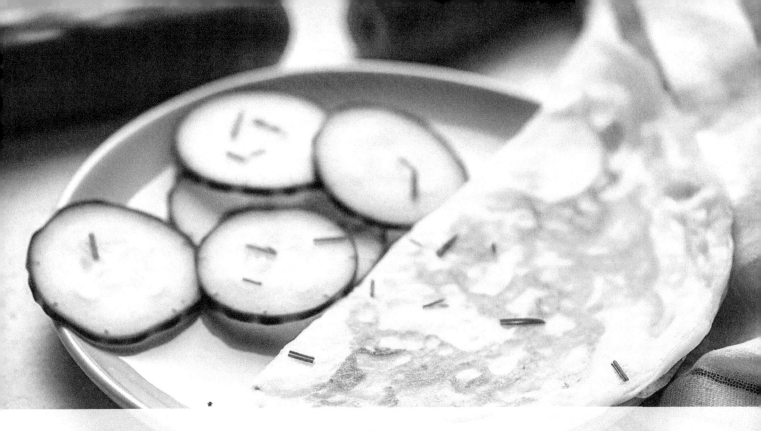

Plain Omelet with Cucumber

 10 Minutes

 1 Serving

INGREDIENTS

- 3 Eggs
- Sea Salt & Black Pepper (to taste)
- 1 tsp Extra Virgin Olive Oil
- ½ Cucumber (medium, sliced)

INSTRUCTIONS

1. Whisk the eggs in a small bowl and season with salt and pepper to taste.

2. Heat the oil in a pan over medium heat. Add the eggs and cook until almost set. Fold in half and transfer the omelet to a plate.

3. Serve with cucumbers and enjoy!

NUTRITION - AMOUNT PER SERVING

Calories	277	Sugar	3g
Fat	19g	Protein	20g
Carbs	7g	Cholesterol	558mg
Fiber	1g	Sodium	216mg

REFER TO PAGE 41 FOR THE ACCOMPANYING TOASTED WALNUT RECIPE

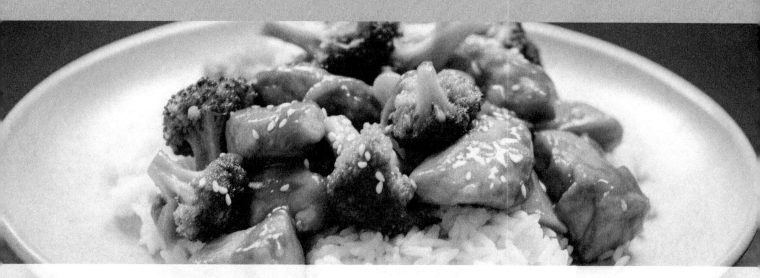

Sweet & Sour Chicken with Broccoli

 20 Minutes   **4 Servings**

INGREDIENTS

- 1 cup Jasmine Rice (dry, rinsed)
- ½ cup Crushed Pineapple
- 3 tbsps Maple Syrup
- 2 tsps Tomato Paste
- 1 tsp Arrowroot Powder
- 1 ½ tbsps Apple Cider Vinegar
- 2 cups Frozen Broccoli Florets
- 1 tbsp Extra Virgin Olive Oil
- 454 grams Chicken Breast (diced)

INSTRUCTIONS

1. Cook the rice according to package directions.
2. Blend the pineapple, maple syrup, tomato paste, arrowroot powder, and apple cider vinegar in a blender. Set aside.
3. Boil the broccoli for 3 – 4 minutes or until tender-crisp.
4. Heat the oil in a pan over medium heat. Add the chicken and cook until browned and cooked through, about 7 to 8 minutes. Add the sauce and the broccoli, and cook for 1 minute or until warmed through. Divide evenly between plates and enjoy!

NUTRITION - AMOUNT PER SERVING

Calories	403	Sugar	14g
Fat	7g	Protein	30g
Carbs	57g	Cholesterol	82mg
Fiber	3g	Sodium	72mg

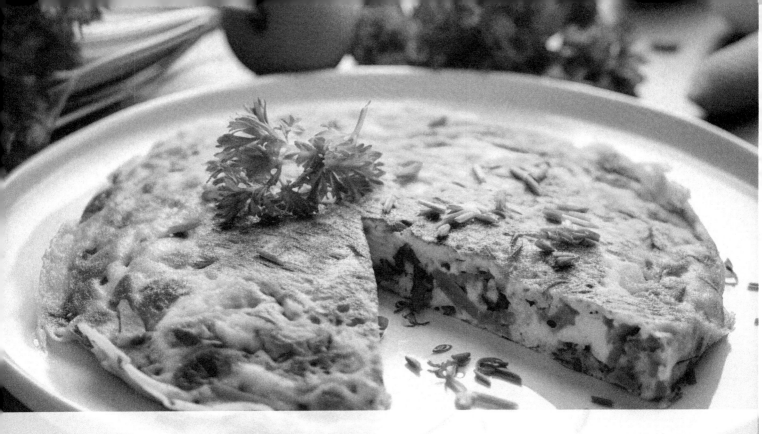

Carrot & Parsley Omelet

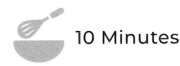 10 Minutes

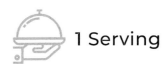 1 Serving

INGREDIENTS

- 1 tsp Butter
- 2 Eggs
- 1 cup Grated Carrot
- 1 tsp Parsley
  (finely chopped)
- Sea Salt & Black Pepper
  (to taste)

INSTRUCTIONS

1. In a non-stick pan, melt the butter over medium heat until it begins to bubble.

2. In a bowl, whisk the eggs. Add the grated carrot and parsley. Mix together and season with salt and pepper to taste.

3. Add the egg mix to the pan. Cook for about 5 minutes or until almost set. Flip the omelet and cook for another 2 to 3 minutes.

4. Remove from heat, plate, and enjoy!

NUTRITION - AMOUNT PER SERVING

Calories	222	Sugar	6g
Fat	14g	Protein	14g
Carbs	11g	Cholesterol	382mg
Fiber	3g	Sodium	219mg

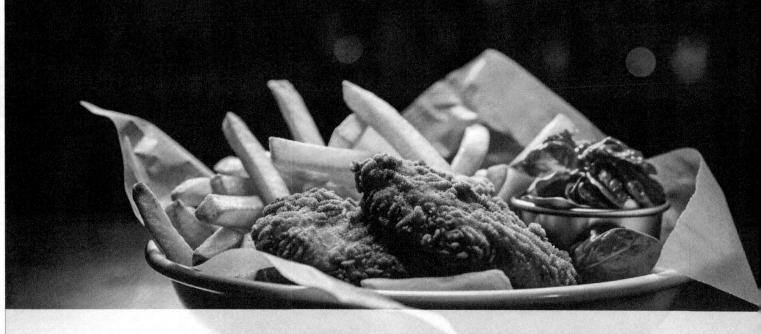

Chicken Fingers & Fries

 40 Minutes

 1 Serving

INGREDIENTS

- 1/4 cup Walnuts
- 1/8 tsp Sea Salt
- 1/8 tsp Black Pepper
- 1/16 tsp Thyme (optional)
- 114 grams Chicken Breast (boneless, skinless)
- 1/2 Yellow Potato (large)
- Sea Salt & Black Pepper (to taste)
- 1 cup Baby Spinach
- 1/3 tsp Apple Cider Vinegar (or balsamic)
- 3/4 tsp Extra Virgin Olive Oil

INSTRUCTIONS

1. Preheat oven to 420°F (216°C) and line a baking sheet with parchment paper.
2. In a food processor, combine walnuts, sea salt, black pepper and thyme. Pulse until it reaches a coarse, sand-like consistency. Add this mixture to a large ziplock bag.
3. Cut your chicken breasts into long pieces and add them to the bag. Shake until the chicken is well coated. Transfer chicken to one side of your baking sheet. Press any extra walnut mix from the bag into the top of the chicken fingers.
4. Slice your potatoes into thin fry-like pieces. Add to a large mixing bowl with a splash of olive oil and season with sea salt and black pepper to taste. Toss until well coated. Transfer them to the baking sheet beside the chicken.
5. Place the baking sheet in the oven and bake for 30 to 40 minutes or until chicken is cooked through and fries are golden brown. Flip the fries at the halfway point.
6. Meanwhile, toss your baby spinach in vinegar and olive oil.
7. Remove chicken and fries from the oven. Plate with the spinach.

NUTRITION - AMOUNT PER SERVING

Calories	453	Sugar	2g
Fat	26g	Protein	33g
Carbs	24g	Cholesterol	83mg
Fiber	5g	Sodium	377mg

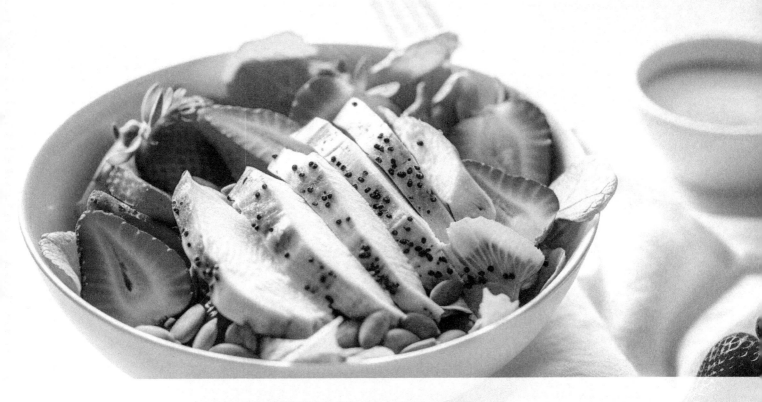

Strawberry Kiwi Salad with Chicken

 5 Minutes

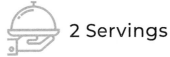 2 Servings

INGREDIENTS

- 1 1/2 tbsps Apple Cider Vinegar
- 1 1/2 tbsps Extra Virgin Olive Oil
- 1 1/2 tsps Maple Syrup
- Sea Salt & Black Pepper (to taste)
- 1 cup Baby Spinach
- 60 grams Strawberries (chopped)
- 2 Kiwi (peeled and chopped)
- 160 grams Chicken Breast, Cooked (sliced)
- 2 tbsps Sunflower Seeds

INSTRUCTIONS

1. In a small bowl combine the apple cider vinegar, oil, and maple syrup. Season with salt and pepper and stir well.

2. Divide the spinach between bowls and top with the chopped strawberries, kiwi, and sunflower seeds. Pour the apple cider vinegar dressing over top and mix well. Top with the chicken and enjoy!

NUTRITION - AMOUNT PER SERVING

Calories	327	Sugar	11g
Fat	17g	Protein	27g
Carbs	18g	Cholesterol	83mg
Fiber	4g	Sodium	55mg

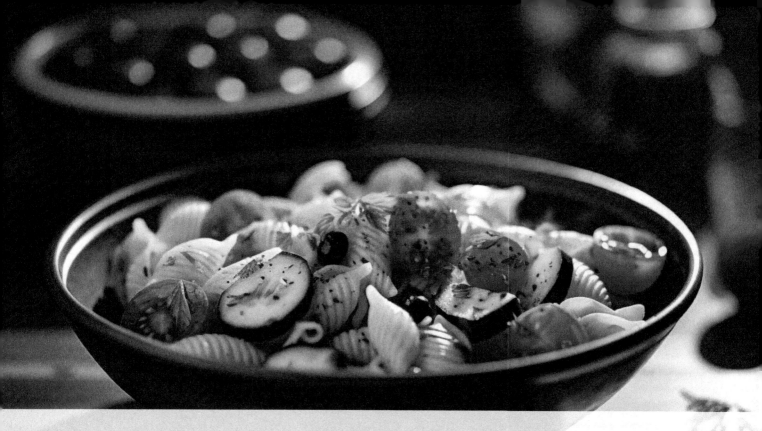

Greek Pasta Salad

 15 minutes

 2 Servings

INGREDIENTS

- ¾ cup Brown Rice Pasta Shells (dry)
- 1 ½ tbsps Extra Virgin Olive Oil
- 2 ¼ tsps Red Wine Vinegar
- ¼ tsp Oregano (dried)
- Sea Salt & Black Pepper (to taste)
- ¾ cup Cherry Tomatoes (halved)
- ¼ Cucumber (quartered, sliced)
- 2 ⅔ tbsps Pitted Kalamata Olives

INSTRUCTIONS

1. Cook the pasta following the instructions on the package. Drain and rinse it thoroughly, then set it aside to cool.

2. In a large bowl, add the oil, red wine vinegar, oregano, salt, and pepper. Mix well to combine.

3. Add the pasta to the dressing and mix well. Add the tomatoes, cucumber, and olives and toss to combine.

NUTRITION - AMOUNT PER SERVING

Calories	292	Sugar	2g
Fat	13g	Protein	5g
Carbs	40g	Cholesterol	0mg
Fiber	3g	Sodium	87mg

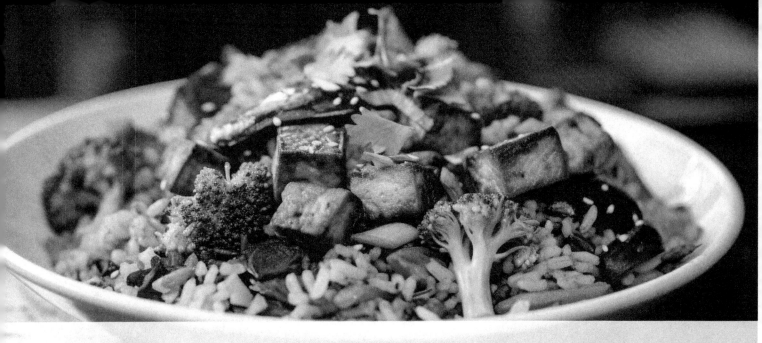

Tofu Veggie Fried Rice

 35 Minutes

 1 Serving

INGREDIENTS

- 1/4 cup Jasmine Rice (uncooked)
- 1 1/8 tsps Sesame Oil (divided)
- 114 grams Tofu (extra firm, drained and diced)
- Sea Salt & Black Pepper
- 1/2 cup Broccoli Florets (chopped)
- 1/4 cup Purple Cabbage (thinly sliced)
- 1/4 Carrot (diced)
- 1 Egg
- 2 1/4 tsps Tamari

INSTRUCTIONS

1. Cook the jasmine rice as per the instructions on the package.
2. Heat half of the sesame oil in a large non-stick pan over medium heat. Cook the tofu for approximately 5 minutes or until it's browned, tossing it frequently. Season with salt and pepper before transferring it to a bowl.
3. Heat the remaining sesame oil over medium heat in the same pan. Cook the broccoli florets, purple cabbage, and carrots until tender, about 5 to 7 minutes.
4. Shift the vegetables to one side of the pan and add the egg to the empty side. Use a spatula to gently move the egg back and forth until scrambled.
5. Place the rice on top of the scrambled egg and use a spatula to break it up. Add the tofu and tamari, then gently stir until everything is thoroughly combined.
6. Transfer to a bowl and enjoy!

NUTRITION - AMOUNT PER SERVING

Calories	407	Sugar	4g
Fat	16g	Protein	24g
Carbs	47g	Cholesterol	186mg
Fiber	4g	Sodium	861mg

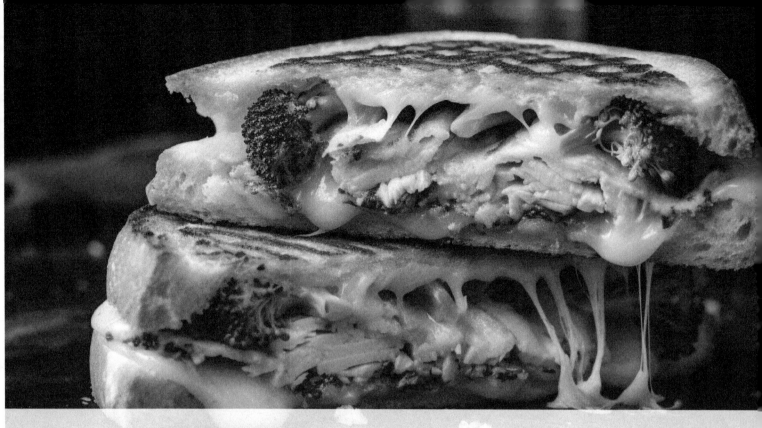

Broccoli, Chicken & Cheese Melt

 15 Minutes

 1 Serving

INGREDIENTS

- 1/2 cup Broccoli Florets (chopped)
- 1 1/2 tsps Butter
- 99 grams Sourdough Bread
- 42 grams Cheddar Cheese (shredded)
- 80 grams Chicken Breast (cooked, shredded)

INSTRUCTIONS

1. Steam the broccoli over a small pot of water for about 5 minutes or until fork tender. Drain and set aside.

2. Heat a skillet over medium-low heat. Spread the butter on the outside of both slices of bread. Add the cooked chicken, the cheddar and broccoli to the middle.

3. Place on the skillet and cook for about 5 minutes per side, until browned on both sides. Remove from the skillet and slice in half.

NUTRITION - AMOUNT PER SERVING

Calories	579	Sugar	1g
Fat	22g	Protein	38g
Carbs	52g	Cholesterol	115mg
Fiber	3g	Sodium	802mg

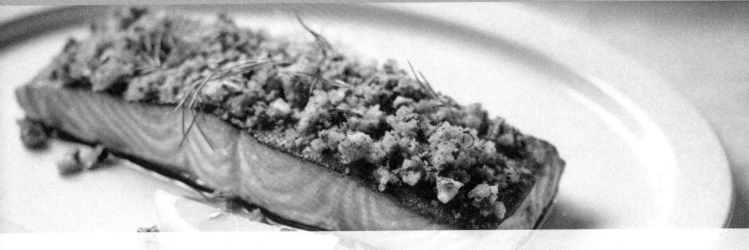

Dinners

Walnut Crusted Salmon

 20 Minutes

 2 Servings

INGREDIENTS

- 1/4 cup Walnuts (very finely chopped)
- 1/4 tsp Sea Salt
- 1/2 tsp Italian Seasoning
- 1/2 tsp Lemon Juice
- 1 tsp Extra Virgin Olive Oil (divided)
- 227 grams Salmon Fillet
- 1/4 Lemon (optional for serving, cut into wedges)

INSTRUCTIONS

1. Preheat the oven to 350°F (176°C) and cover a baking sheet with parchment paper.

2. Combine the walnuts, salt and Italian seasoning. Stir in the lemon juice and half of the oil.

3. Rub the remaining oil evenly over all sides of the salmon fillet(s). Place the salmon fillet(s) onto the baking sheet, skin side facing down. Spoon the walnut mixture onto the top side of the salmon and gently press it down using the back of a spoon to ensure the walnut mixture remains in place.

4. Bake for about 12 to 15 minutes until the salmon is cooked and flakes easily. Plate and serve with lemon wedges.

NUTRITION - AMOUNT PER SERVING

Calories	267	Sugar	0g
Fat	17g	Protein	28g
Carbs	2g	Cholesterol	58mg
Fiber	1g	Sodium	384mg

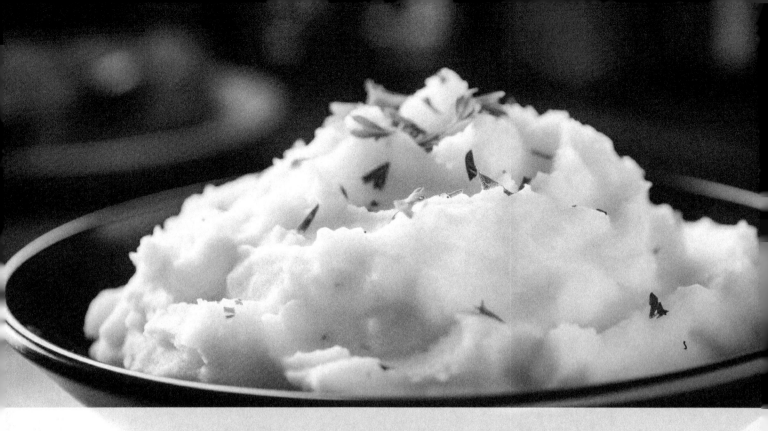

Mashed Potatoes

 20 minutes

 2 Servings

INGREDIENTS

- ¾ tsp Sea Salt (divided)
- 2 Russet Potatoes (medium, peeled and chopped)
- 2 tsps Butter

INSTRUCTIONS

1. Bring a large pot of water to a boil. Add ½ of the salt to the water.
2. Place the chopped potatoes into the water and boil for about 12 - 15 minutes until soft.
3. Drain the water, add butter, and using a potato masher, mash until creamy. Season with the remaining salt to taste.
4. Divide onto plates with another protein or side(s).

NUTRITION - AMOUNT PER SERVING

Calories	164	Sugar	2g
Fat	0g	Protein	5g
Carbs	37g	Cholesterol	0mg
Fiber	4g	Sodium	909mg

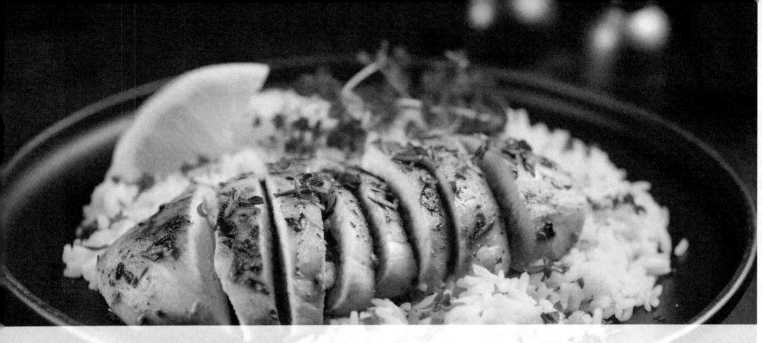

Maple Dijon Chicken & Lemon Herb Rice

 50 Minutes

 2 Servings

INGREDIENTS

- 1 tbsp dijon Mustard
- 1 tbsp Maple Syrup
- 1 1/2 tbsps Lemon Juice (divided)
- 1/2 tsp Oregano (dried, divided)
- 1/4 tsp Sea Salt (divided)
- 227 grams Chicken Breast
- 3/4 cup Water
- 1/2 tsp Dried Basil
- 1/2 cup Jasmine Rice

INSTRUCTIONS

1. In a shallow bowl or zipper-lock bag combine the Dijon mustard, maple syrup, ⅓ of the lemon juice, half of the oregano, and half of the salt. Reserve a quarter of the marinade for later. Add the chicken to the remaining marinade and let it marinate for at least 20 minutes.

2. Preheat the oven to 375°F (190°C).

3. Transfer the chicken and the marinade to a baking dish and bake for 25 to 30 minutes or until the chicken is cooked through. Brush the chicken generously with the reserved marinade.

4. Meanwhile, make the rice by heating the water in a pot over medium-high heat. Add the basil, remaining oregano, and the remaining salt. Bring to a boil then stir in the rice. Cover with a lid, reduce heat to low and cook the rice for 10 to 12 minutes or until the liquid is absorbed and the rice is tender.

5. Remove the rice from the heat, stir in the remaining lemon juice and let the rice rest covered for about five minutes. Fluff with a fork and season with additional lemon juice or salt if needed. To serve, divide the chicken and rice between plates and enjoy!

NUTRITION - AMOUNT PER SERVING

Calories	333	Sugar	6g
Fat	3g	Protein	29g
Carbs	46g	Cholesterol	83mg
Fiber	1g	Sodium	432mg

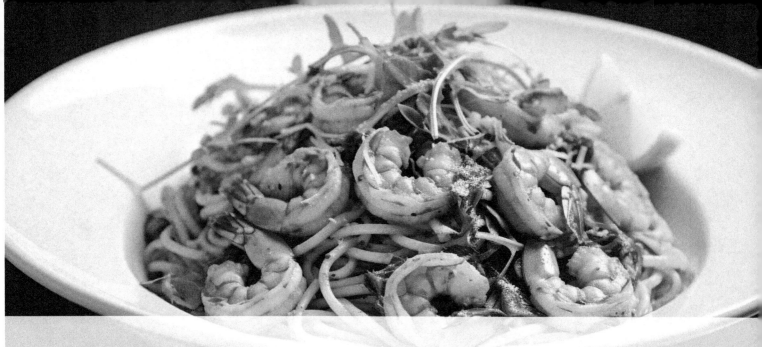

Lemony Shrimp Pasta

 20 Minutes

 1 Serving

INGREDIENTS

- ¼ cup Brown Rice Spaghetti
- 1 tbsp Butter (divided)
- 1 tbsp Extra Virgin Olive Oil (divided)
- 114 grams Shrimp (peeled, deveined)
- 1 cup Arugula
- 1 tbsp Lemon Juice
- Sea Salt & Black Pepper (to taste)

INSTRUCTIONS

1. Prepare the spaghetti following the instructions on the package. Once cooked, remove it from the heat, strain, and rinse with cold water to prevent overcooking.

2. Melt half the butter in a skillet over medium heat. Add the extra virgin olive oil and cook the shrimp for 1 to 3 minutes on each side or until they are no longer translucent. Set the cooked shrimp aside. Then, add the arugula to the skillet and sauté it until it just wilts.

3. Combine the pasta with the shrimp in the pan, then add the lemon juice and the remaining butter and olive oil. Toss everything together to coat evenly. Divide the dish onto plates and season with salt and pepper to taste.

NUTRITION - AMOUNT PER SERVING

Calories	526	Sugar	1g
Fat	27g	Protein	28g
Carbs	45g	Cholesterol	213mg
Fiber	2g	Sodium	142mg

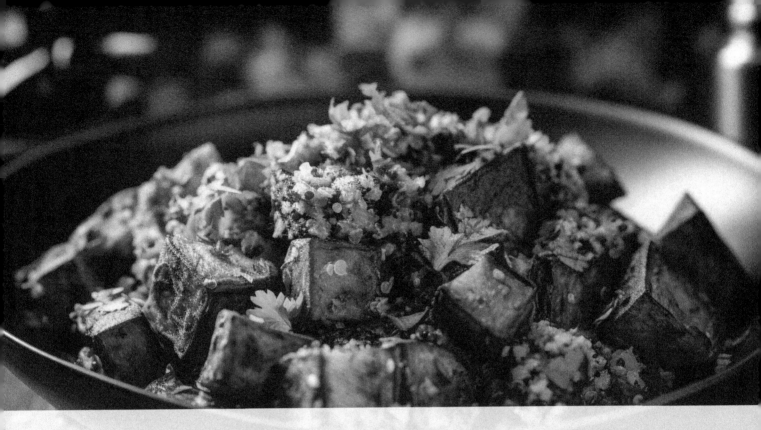

Marinated Eggplant with Quinoa

 30 Minutes

 3 Servings

INGREDIENTS

- 75 grams Eggplant (stem removed, cubed)
- 1/3 cup Water
- 1 1/2 tbsps Tamari
- 2 1/4 tsps Rice Vinegar
- 3/4 tsp Maple Syrup
- 3/4 cup Quinoa (dry, uncooked)
- 3 tbsps Cilantro (finely chopped)

INSTRUCTIONS

1. Preheat the oven to 450°F (232°C).

2. In a baking dish, combine the eggplant, water, tamari, rice vinegar and maple syrup until well coated. Roast for 30 minutes or until golden brown, stirring halfway.

3. Meanwhile, cook the quinoa according to package instructions.

4. Divide the quinoa onto plates and top with the roasted eggplant. Garnish with cilantro and enjoy!

NUTRITION - AMOUNT PER SERVING

Calories	173	Sugar	2g
Fat	3g	Protein	7g
Carbs	30g	Cholesterol	0mg
Fiber	4g	Sodium	507mg

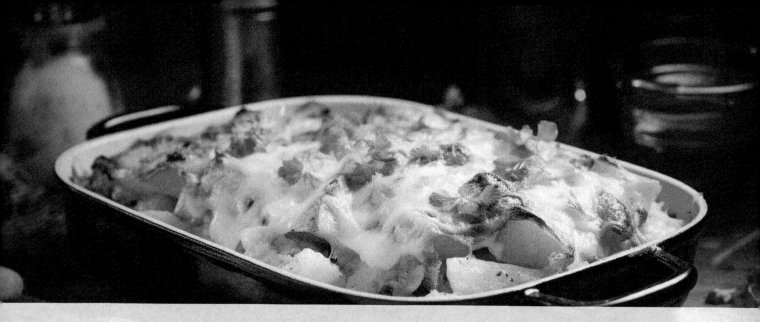

Chicken & Potato Casserole

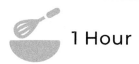 1 Hour

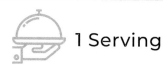 1 Serving

INGREDIENTS

- 1/2 tsp Extra Virgin Olive Oil (divided)
- 113 grams Extra Lean Ground Chicken
- 1/16 tsp Sea Salt (divided)
- 1/3 Russet Potato (peeled, shredded, squeezed and drained of excess liquid)
- 1/4 cup Unsweetened Almond Milk
- 2 Eggs
- 1/16 tsp Oregano
- 28 grams Cheddar Cheese (shredded)

INSTRUCTIONS

1. Preheat the oven to 400°F (205C). Grease a baking dish with half the oil.

2. Over medium-high heat, heat the remaining oil in a pan before adding the ground chicken. Use a spoon to break up the chicken as it cooks. Drain any excess liquid, season with half of the salt, and transfer to the baking dish.

3. Sprinkle the shredded potato evenly over the cooked chicken.

4. In a bowl, whisk together the almond milk, eggs, oregano, and the remaining salt. Pour the mixture over all the ingredients in the baking dish. Then, sprinkle the cheese over top and bake for about 45 minutes until cooked and golden brown.

5. Let it cool slightly before cutting into squares.

NUTRITION - AMOUNT PER SERVING

Calories	406	Sugar	1g
Fat	25g	Protein	32g
Carbs	14g	Cholesterol	250mg
Fiber	2g	Sodium	447mg

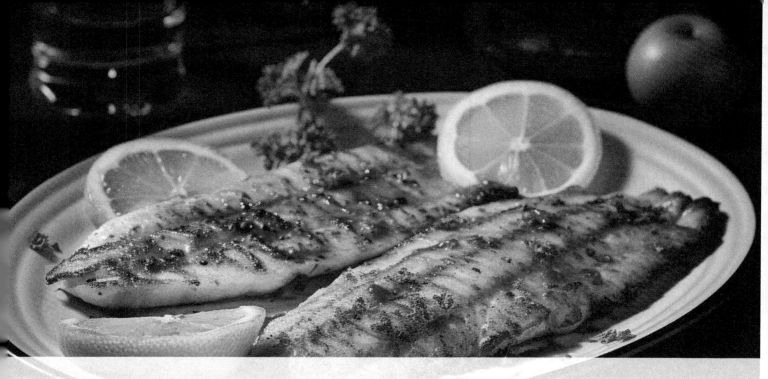

Broiled Lemon & Pepper Sole

 10 Minutes

 2 Servings

INGREDIENTS

- 1 tsp Avocado Oil
- 1/4 tsp Paprika
- 1/4 tsp Black Pepper
- 1/4 tsp Chili Powder
- 1/8 tsp Sea Salt
- 227 grams Sole Fillet
- 1/4 Lemon (juiced)

INSTRUCTIONS

1. Preheat the broiler to high and move the rack to the top rung. Lightly grease a baking sheet with some of the oil.
2. In a small bowl combine the paprika, black pepper, chili powder, and salt.
3. Pat the fillets dry with a paper towel. Place on the prepared baking sheet and drizzle with the remaining oil. Season the fillets with the paprika mixture and use the back of a spoon to evenly coat each fillet with the oil and spices.
4. Broil the fillets for 3 to 4 minutes or until cooked through and the fillets flake easily. (Cooking time may vary depending on the thickness of the fillets.)
5. Drizzle with the lemon juice then divide between plates.

NUTRITION - AMOUNT PER SERVING

Calories	104	Sugar	10g
Fat	5g	Protein	14g
Carbs	1g	Cholesterol	51mg
Fiber	0g	Sodium	493mg

REFER TO PAGE 57 FOR THE ACCOMPANYING QUINOA RECIPE

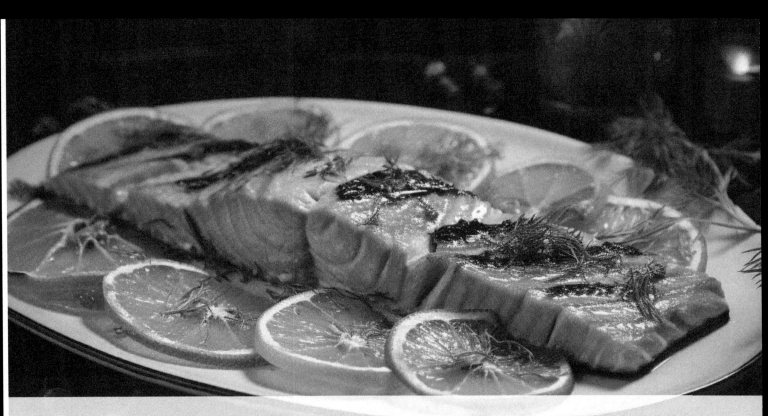

Slow Roasted Salmon with Citrus

 40 Minutes

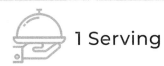 1 Serving

INGREDIENTS

- 1/8 bulb Fennel (cored, thinly sliced)
- 1/4 Navel Orange (thinly sliced)
- 1/4 Lemon (thinly sliced)
- 1/16 tsp Sea Salt (divided)
- 113 grams Salmon Fillet
- 1 tbsp Extra Virgin Olive Oil
- 1 tbsp Parsley (finely chopped)

INSTRUCTIONS

1. Preheat the oven to 300°F (149°C).

2. Add the fennel, orange, lemon, and half the sea salt to an oven-safe baking dish and mix to combine. Rest the salmon on top, season with the remaining salt, and drizzle with extra virgin olive oil. Place the dish in the oven for 30 to 35 minutes or until the salmon reaches your preferred level of doneness.

3. Remove from the oven, plate, and top with parsley.

NUTRITION - AMOUNT PER SERVING

Calories	298	Sugar	4g
Fat	19g	Protein	26g
Carbs	8g	Cholesterol	58mg
Fiber	2g	Sodium	254mg

REFER TO PAGE 63 FOR THE ACCOMPANYING BAKED POTATO RECIPE

Snacks

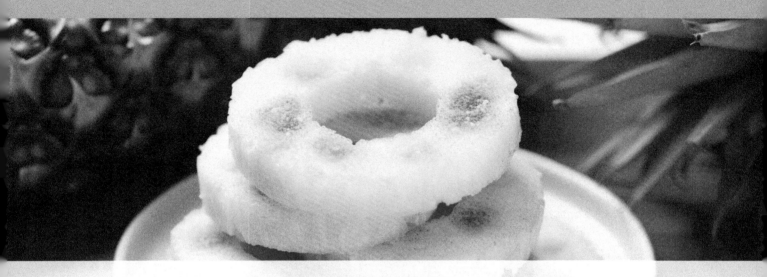

Pineapple with Cinnamon

 5 Minutes

 2 Servings

INGREDIENTS

- 2 cups Pineapple (cored and sliced into rounds)
- 1 tsp Cinnamon

INSTRUCTIONS

1. Put pineapple on a plate and sprinkle with cinnamon.
2. Serve and enjoy!

NUTRITION - AMOUNT PER SERVING

Calories	86	Sugar	16g
Fat	0g	Protein	1g
Carbs	23g	Cholesterol	0mg
Fiber	3g	Sodium	2mg

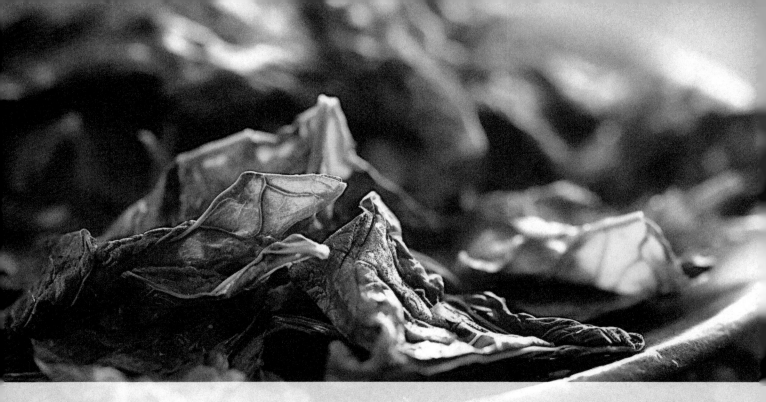

Sea Salt Spinach Chips

 30 Minutes

 2 Servings

INGREDIENTS

- 1 cup Baby Spinach
- 2 tsps Avocado Oil
- 1/8 tsp Sea Salt (or to taste)

INSTRUCTIONS

1. Preheat the oven to 300°F (150°C) and line a large baking sheet with parchment paper.

2. Place the spinach in a mixing bowl and drizzle with the oil. Use your hands to mix the spinach and lightly coat each leaf with the oil. Add the salt and mix again to season the leaves evenly.

3. In batches, arrange the spinach leaves on the baking sheet in an even layer being careful not to overcrowd the baking sheet. Season with additional salt, if desired. Bake for 12 to 15 minutes or until the leaves are dry and crispy.

4. Transfer to a plate and repeat with remaining spinach.

NUTRITION - AMOUNT PER SERVING

Calories	43	Sugar	0g
Fat	5g	Protein	0g
Carbs	1g	Cholesterol	0mg
Fiber	0g	Sodium	159mg

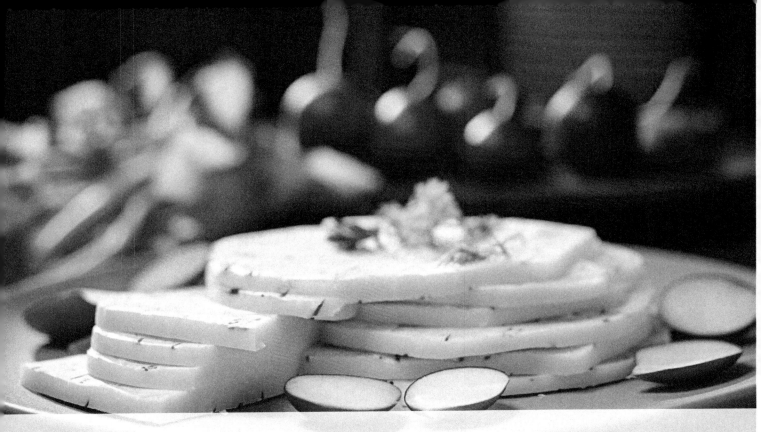

Radishes & Swiss Cheese

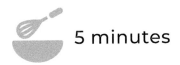 5 minutes

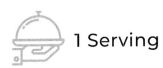 1 Serving

INGREDIENTS

- 1 cup Radishes
- 45 grams Swiss Cheese (sliced)

INSTRUCTIONS

1. Serve the radishes with the cheese.

NUTRITION - AMOUNT PER SERVING

Calories	195	Sugar	2g
Fat	14g	Protein	13g
Carbs	5g	Cholesterol	42mg
Fiber	2g	Sodium	129mg

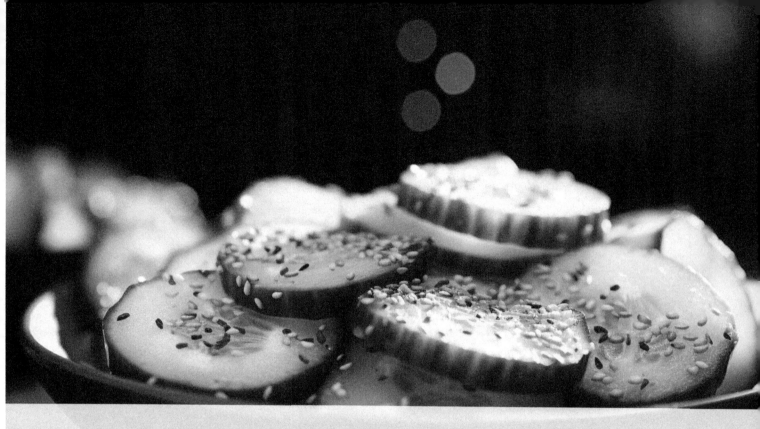

Sesame Cucumber Salad

 5 Minutes

 2 Servings

INGREDIENTS

- 2 tbsps Rice Vinegar
- 1 tbsp Maple Syrup
- 1/2 tsp Tamari
- 1 Cucumber (peeled, chopped)
- 1 tsp Sesame Seeds (black or white, toasted)

INSTRUCTIONS

1. In a bowl, whisk together the rice vinegar, maple syrup and tamari.
2. Add the cucumber and toss until well coated.
3. Garnish with sesame seeds and enjoy!

NUTRITION - AMOUNT PER SERVING

Calories	58	Sugar	9g
Fat	1g	Protein	1g
Carbs	13g	Cholesterol	0mg
Fiber	1g	Sodium	88mg

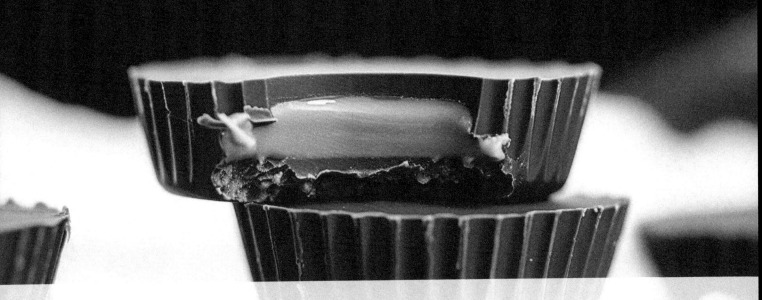

Dark Chocolate Peanut Butter Cups

 1 Hour 15 Minutes

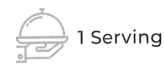 1 Serving

INGREDIENTS

- 15 grams Dark Chocolate (at least 70% cacao, broken into pieces)
- 1/2 tsp Coconut Oil
- 2 1/3 tsps All Natural Peanut Butter
- 1/16 tsp Vanilla Extract
- 1/16 tsp Sea Salt

INSTRUCTIONS

1. Position paper baking cups on a plate or small baking sheet.
2. Create a double boiler by filling a medium pot with an inch of water. Place a smaller pot or heat-safe bowl on top without letting water touch it. Make sure it sits securely, allowing no water or steam to escape. Bring the water to a boil and then lower the heat to its lowest setting.
3. Use the double boiler: Bring the water to a boil, then reduce the heat to its lowest setting. Place dark chocolate and coconut oil in the smaller pot, stirring until fully melted. Remove from heat.
4. Fill half of the paper baking cups with the melted chocolate, ensuring an even, thin layer in each. Freeze for 10 to 15 minutes until solid.
5. Mix peanut butter, vanilla, and salt in a bowl while they freeze. Stir until smooth.
6. Spoon peanut butter onto the center of the solid chocolate in each baking cup. Drizzle the remaining dark chocolate around and over the peanut butter.
7. Return to the freezer for approximately 30 minutes or until solid.

NUTRITION - AMOUNT PER SERVING

Calories	186	Sugar	5g
Fat	15g	Protein	4g
Carbs	10g	Cholesterol	0mg
Fiber	2g	Sodium	35mg

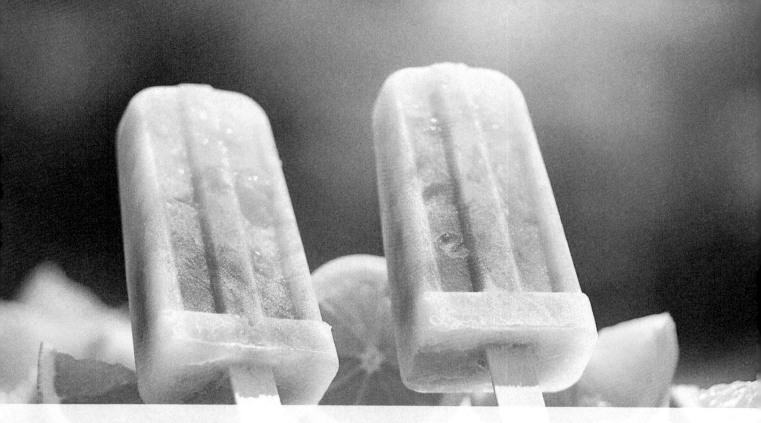

Orange Popsicles

 5 Hours

 5 Servings

INGREDIENTS

- 1 Carrot (small, peeled and chopped)
- 1 ½ cups Orange Juice (freshly squeezed)
- 2 tbsps Maple Syrup

INSTRUCTIONS

1. Add the carrots to a small pot of boiling water. Cook for 8 to 10 minutes or until very tender. Drain and rinse the cooked carrots with cold water to help them cool. Set aside.

2. Add the orange juice, maple syrup, and cooked carrots to a blender and blend until very smooth and creamy.

3. Carefully pour the orange juice mixture into a popsicle mold and transfer to the freezer.

4. Freeze for about 60 minutes or until partially frozen. Insert popsicle sticks. Allow the popsicles to chill in the freezer for four to five hours more or until solid.

NUTRITION - AMOUNT PER SERVING

Calories	159	Sugar	12g
Fat	0g	Protein	1g
Carbs	14g	Cholesterol	0mg
Fiber	0g	Sodium	10mg

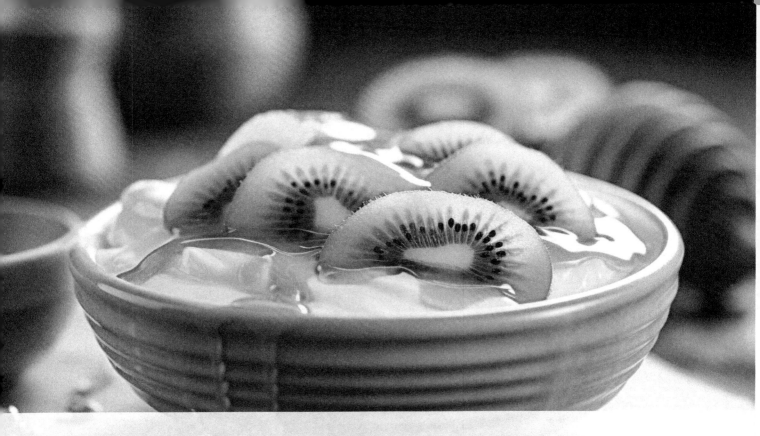

Kiwi, Yogurt & Maple Syrup

 5 Minutes

 1 Serving

INGREDIENTS

- 1/2 cup Unsweetened Coconut Yogurt
- 1 Kiwi (peeled and sliced)
- 1 tsp Maple Syrup (optional)

INSTRUCTIONS

1. Add the yogurt and kiwi to a bowl.
2. Top with maple syrup, if using. Enjoy!

NUTRITION - AMOUNT PER SERVING

Calories	115	Sugar	11g
Fat	4g	Protein	1g
Carbs	21g	Cholesterol	0mg
Fiber	4g	Sodium	28mg

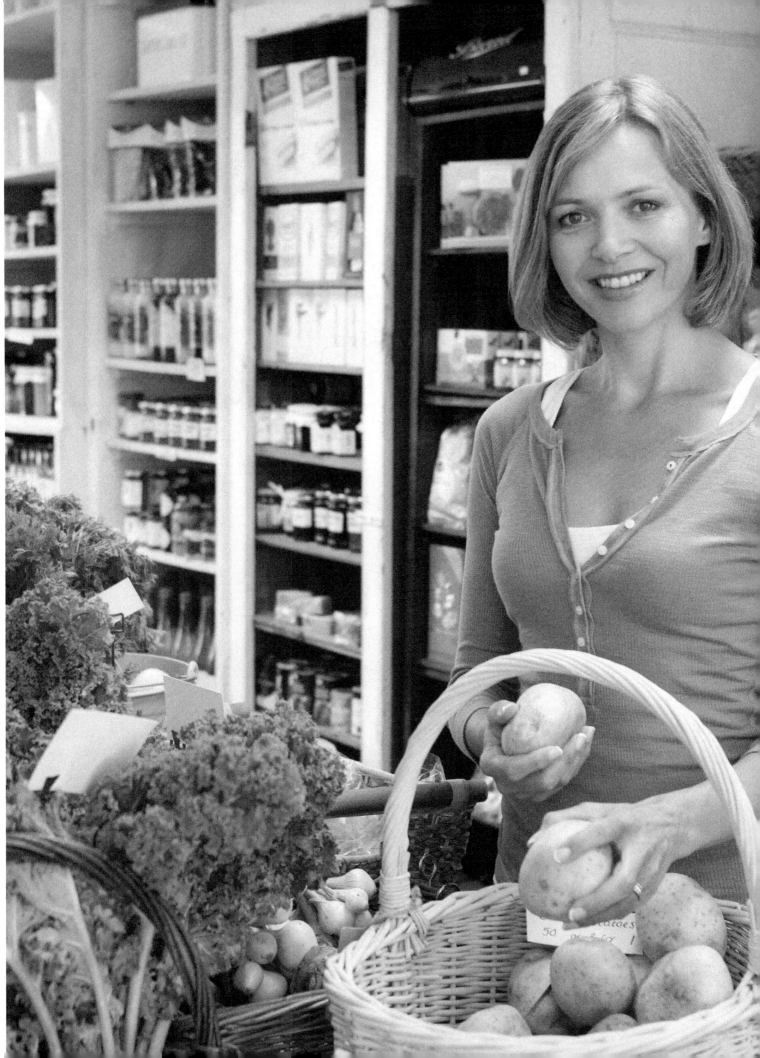

WEEK 4

'7-Days Meal Plan

MONDAY

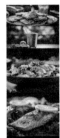

BREAKFAST
Coconut Plantain Pancakes, Kiwi Green Smoothie

LUNCH
Creamy Dill Salad with Chicken

DINNER
Massaged Kale Salad with Salmon

SNACKS
Papaya with Yogurt & Walnuts

TUESDAY

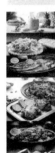

BREAKFAST
Warm Parsley Tomato Plantain Wrap

LUNCH
 Spinach Tuna Crepes

DINNER
Potato Shepherd's Pie

SNACKS
Frozen Coconut Yogurt Covered Strawberries

WEDNESDAY

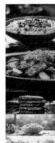

BREAKFAST
Coconut Matcha Smoothie, Tuna Rice Cake

LUNCH
Broiled Mackerel, Curried Kale Salad

DINNER
Baked Cilantro Lime Chicken , Tomato & Thyme Quinoa

SNACKS
Kiwi & Strawberries

THURSDAY

BREAKFAST
Maple Walnut Millet Porridge

LUNCH
Cajun Chicken, Potatoes & Kale

DINNER
Maple Beef Burgers, Herbed Rice

SNACKS
Lemon Dill Yogurt Dip & Carrots

FRIDAY

BREAKFAST
Steak & Potato Egg Mffns

LUNCH
Grilled Tempeh & Eggplant with Rice

DINNER
Zucchini & Tuna Pasta Salad

SNACKS
Orange & Strawberry Frozen Yogurt Bites

SATURDAY

BREAKFAST
Turmeric Quinoa Breakfast Bowls

LUNCH
Pan Fried Tofu Spinach Salad

DINNER
Cumin Roasted Chicken & Broccoli

SNACKS
Cucumbers & Salmon Dip

SUNDAY

BREAKFAST
Orange Creamsicle Chia Pudding, Pumpkin Seeds Cup

LUNCH
Meatball Lettuce Wraps

DINNER
Pan-Fried Trout with Herbed Rice

SNACKS
Brazilian Cheese Bread

Shopping List

FRUITS

2 Kiwi
1 ¼ Lemon
⅓ cup Lemon Juice
1 Lime
1 ½ tbsps Lime Juice
1 ⅓ Navel Orange
1 cup Papaya
1 cup Pineapple
1 ⅔ Plantain
3 ¼ tbsps Strawberries
120 grams Strawberries

SEEDS, NUTS & SPICES

1 tbsp Cajun Spice
2 ¾ tbsps Chia Seeds
⅛ tsp Cinnamon
2 ¼ tsps Cumin Seed
1 ½ tsps Curry Powder
¼ tsp Dried Thyme
¾ tsp Fennel Seed
½ tsp Ground Sage
2 tbsps Hemp Seeds
1 ½ tsps Italian Seasoning
½ tsp Oregano
⅓ cup Pumpkin Seeds
Sea Salt & Black Pepper
½ tsp Turmeric
¾ cup Walnuts

FROZEN

2 Ice Cubes

VEGETABLES

1 ½ cups Baby Carrots
5 ¼ cups Baby Spinach
1 head Boston Lettuce
75 grams Broccoli
1 ½ Carrots
2 cups Cherry Tomatoes
2 tbsps Cilantro
1 Cucumber

⅓ Eggplant
⅔ cup Fresh Dill
1 tsp Ginger
¾ cup Grated Carrot
2 cups Kale Leaves
225 grams Kale Leaves
⅔ cup Parsley
2 leaves Romaine
½ head Romaine Hearts
¾ tsp Thyme
2 ¼ Yellow Potato
65 grams Zucchini

PANTRY STAPLES

¾ cup Basmati Rice
¼ cup Brown Basmati Rice
¼ cup Brown Rice
½ cup Brown Rice Macaroni
½ cup Canned Coconut Milk
107 grams Canned Wild
   Salmon
2 ⅔ tbsps Millet
¾ cups Quinoa
3 cans Tuna
1 ½ cups Vegetable Broth,
   Low Sodium
1 tsp Green Tea Powder
3 ½ tbsps Maple Syrup
2 Plain Rice Cake

BAKING

1 cup Brown Rice Flour
¼ cup Tapioca Flour
1 ⅓ tsps Vanilla Extract

BREAD, FISH, MEAT & CHEESE

263 grams Chicken Breast
113 grams Chicken Thighs
553 grams Extra Lean
   Ground Beef
227 grams Extra Lean
   Ground Chicken
113 grams Mackerel Fillet
2 ⅔ tbsps Parmigiano
   Reggiano
1 Rainbow Trout Fillet
160 grams Salmon Fillet
113 grams Tempeh
200 grams Tofu
114 grams Top Sirloin Steak

CONDIMENTS & OILS

1 ½ tbsps Apple Cider
   Vinegar
2 ½ tbsps Avocado Oil
½ cup Black Olives
1 tbsp Coconut Aminos
2 1/16 tbsps Coconut Oil
½ cupExtra Virgin Olive Oil
⅔ tsp Sesame Oil
2 tbsps Tahini
2 ⅛ tbsps Tamari

FRIDGE

1 ½ tbsps Butter
11 Eggs
2 tbsps Orange Juice
3 cups Unsweetened
   Almond Milk
2 ½ cups Unsweetened
   Coconut Yogurt

Breakfasts

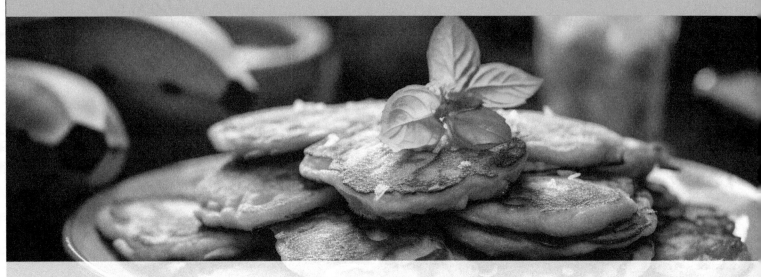

Coconut Plantain Pancakes

 20 Minutes

 1 Serving

INGREDIENTS

- ⅔ Plantain (ripe, peeled)
- 2 Eggs
- ⅛ tsp Sea Salt
- ¼ cup Brown Rice Flour
- 2 tsps Coconut Oil

INSTRUCTIONS

1. In a blender, combine the plantain, eggs and salt. Slowly add the flour until everything is well combined.
2. Over medium heat, heat coconut oil in a skillet. Use the batter to make 4 small pancakes, cooking for approximately 1 to 2 minutes on each side.
3. Serve pancakes with your choice of toppings and enjoy!

NUTRITION - AMOUNT PER SERVING

Calories	491	Sugar	32g
Fat	14g	Protein	9g
Carbs	88g	Cholesterol	124mg
Fiber	5g	Sodium	353mg

156

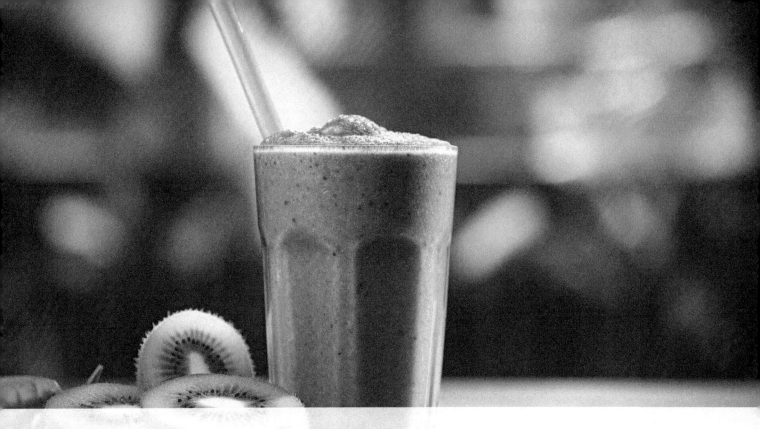

Kiwi Green Smoothie

 5 Minutes

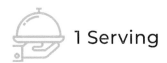 1 Serving

INGREDIENTS

- 1 Kiwi (small, peeled)
- 1 tbsp Chia Seeds
- 1 1/4 cups Baby Spinach
- 1 cup Water
- 2 Ice Cubes

INSTRUCTIONS

1. Place all ingredients in your blender and blend until smooth.

2. Pour into a glass and enjoy!

NUTRITION - AMOUNT PER SERVING

Calories	107	Sugar	6g
Fat	4g	Protein	4g
Carbs	16g	Cholesterol	0mg
Fiber	7g	Sodium	38mg

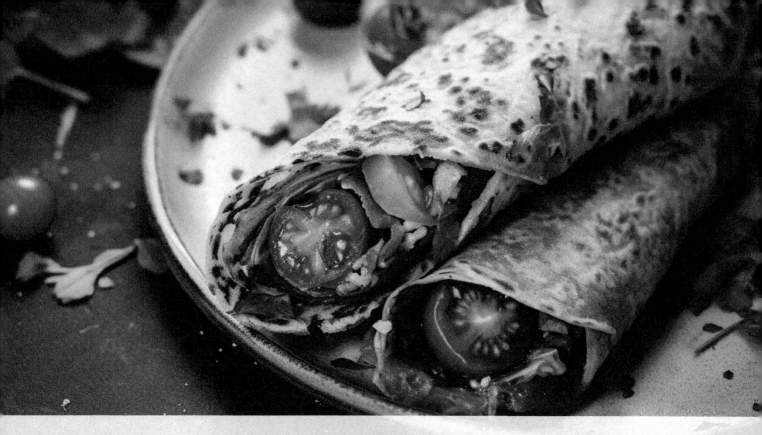

Warm Parsley Tomato Plantain Wrap

 15 Minutes

 2 Servings

INGREDIENTS

- 1 Plantain (very ripe, mashed)
- 1 Egg
- 1 1/2 tsps Parsley (chopped)
- 3/4 cup Cherry Tomatoes (halved)

INSTRUCTIONS

1. Preheat the oven to 375°F (190°C). Line a baking sheet with parchment paper or a silicone baking mat.

2. In a bowl, stir together the mashed plantain and egg. Transfer to the baking sheet, spreading thinly to form circles of approximately 4 to 5 inches wide. Bake for 10 minutes or until cooked through and golden brown.

3. Transfer each wrap to a plate and fill with the parsley and tomatoes.

NUTRITION - AMOUNT PER SERVING

Calories	211	Sugar	25g
Fat	3g	Protein	5g
Carbs	45g	Cholesterol	93mg
Fiber	3g	Sodium	44mg

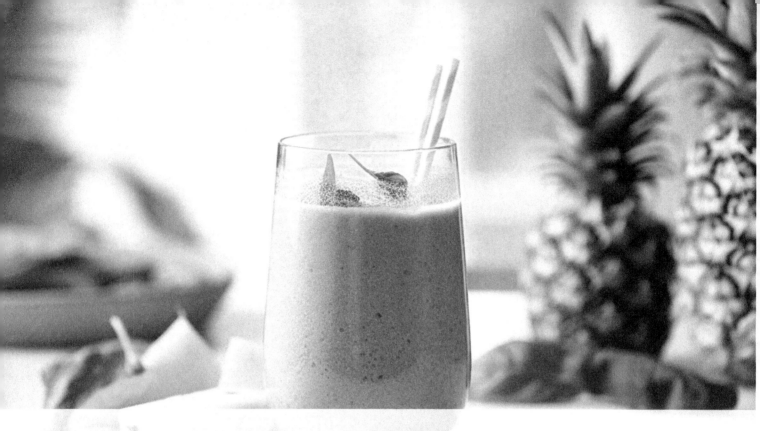

Coconut Matcha Smoothie

 5 Minutes

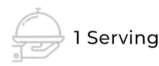 1 Serving

INGREDIENTS

- ¾ cup Unsweetened Almond Milk
- 1 cup Pineapple
- 1 cup Baby Spinach
- 1 tbsp Hemp Seeds
- 1 tsp Green Tea Powder (matcha)

INSTRUCTIONS

1. Place all ingredients together in a blender.
2. Blend until smooth.
3. Pour into a glass and enjoy!

NUTRITION - AMOUNT PER SERVING

Calories	166	Sugar	17g
Fat	7g	Protein	6g
Carbs	24g	Cholesterol	0mg
Fiber	4g	Sodium	146mg

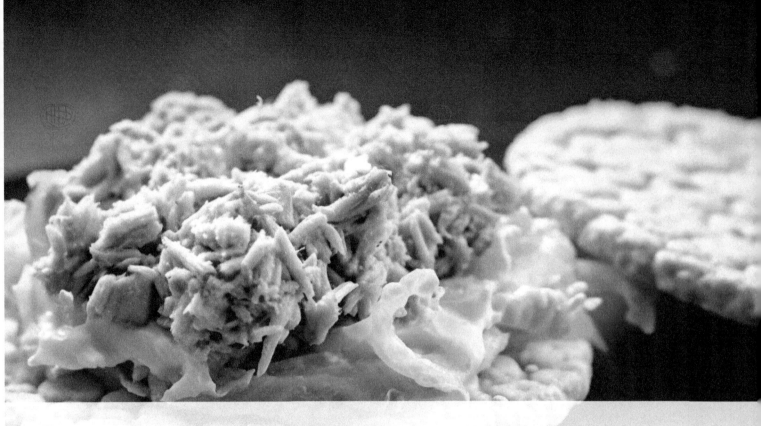

Tuna Rice Cake

 5 Minutes

 2 Servings

INGREDIENTS

- 1 can Tuna (drained)
- Sea Salt & Black Pepper (to taste)
- 2 Plain Rice Cakes
- 2 leaves Romaine Lettuce

INSTRUCTIONS

1. Mash the tuna with a fork in a bowl, season with salt and pepper.
2. Top the rice cakes with the lettuce and then the tuna mixture.

NUTRITION - AMOUNT PER SERVING

Calories	111	Sugar	0g
Fat	1g	Protein	17g
Carbs	8g	Cholesterol	30mg
Fiber	1g	Sodium	208mg

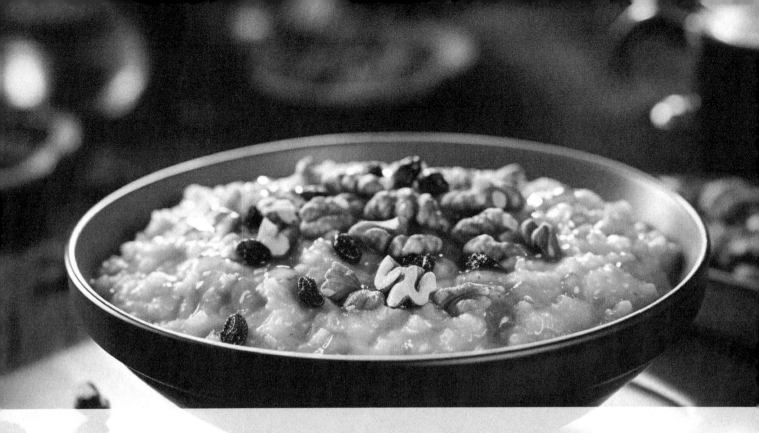

Maple Walnut Millet Porridge

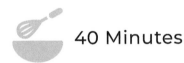 40 Minutes

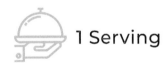 1 Serving

INGREDIENTS

- 1 cup Unsweetened Almond Milk
- 2 ⅔ tbsps Millet (uncooked)
- 1 tbsp Maple Syrup (divided)
- ⅔ tsp Vanilla Extract
- ¼ cup Walnuts (chopped)

INSTRUCTIONS

1. Combine the almond milk, millet, ⅔ of the maple syrup and vanilla in a large pot over medium-high heat. Bring to a gentle boil then reduce the heat to low and cover the pot with a lid. Let it simmer for 30 to 35 minutes, or until the millet is tender and your desired consistency is reached. Be sure to stir occasionally.

2. Remove from the heat and stir in the remaining maple syrup. Serve in a bowl topped with walnuts.

NUTRITION - AMOUNT PER SERVING

Calories	411	Sugar	13g
Fat	23g	Protein	9g
Carbs	43g	Cholesterol	0mg
Fiber	6g	Sodium	166mg

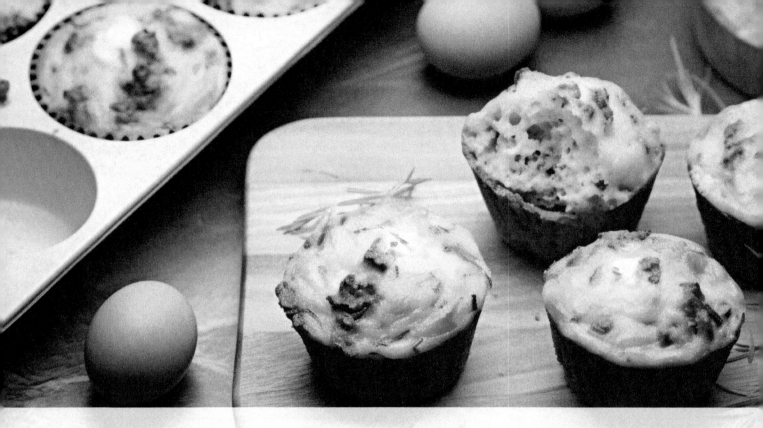

Steak & Potato Egg Muffins

 45 Minutes

 1 Serving

INGREDIENTS

- 1/2 tsp Extra Virgin Olive Oil
- 114 grams Top Sirloin Steak
- 2 Eggs (whisked)
- 1/4 Yellow Potato (medium, chopped into small cubes)
- Sea Salt & Black Pepper (to taste)

INSTRUCTIONS

1. Preheat the oven to 375°F (190°C). Line a muffin tray with paper liners or use a silicone tray.

2. Heat the oil in a pan over medium heat. Add the steak and cook for 5 minutes on each side, or until desired doneness. Slice into small pieces.

3. Add the eggs, steak, potato, salt, and pepper to a bowl. Stir to combine. Divide the mixture evenly between muffin cups.

4. Bake in the oven for 30 minutes, or until they have risen and started to brown on the top.

NUTRITION - AMOUNT PER SERVING

Calories	518	Sugar	1g
Fat	33g	Protein	43g
Carbs	10g	Cholesterol	647mg
Fiber	1g	Sodium	274mg

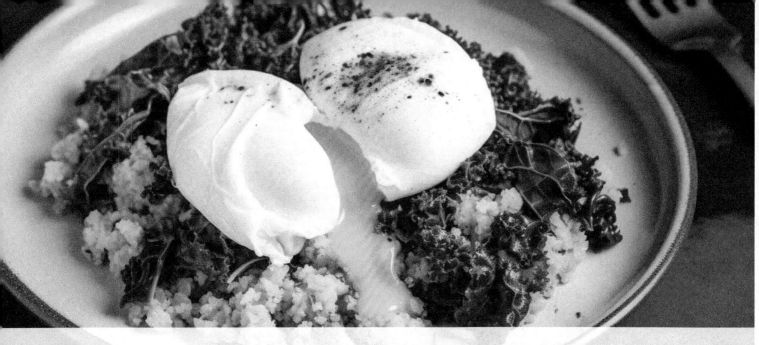

Turmeric Quinoa Breakfast Bowls

 20 Minutes   2 Servings

INGREDIENTS

- 1/2 cup Quinoa (dry)
- 1/2 tsp Turmeric
- 1/4 tsp Sea Salt
- 1 tsp Ginger (fresh, grated or minced)
- 1 tbsp Lime Juice (divided)
- 1 tbsp Apple Cider Vinegar
- 4 Eggs
- 2 cups Kale Leaves (finely chopped)
- 2 tbsps Water

INSTRUCTIONS

1. Combine quinoa, turmeric, salt, ginger, and half of the lime juice in a pot. Cook the quinoa following the package instructions. Once cooked, mix in the remaining lime juice.

2. In a separate pot, boil water, then add vinegar. Create a whirlpool by stirring the water with a spoon. Gently add the eggs to the water, working in batches if necessary to avoid overcrowding. Cook for 3 to 4 minutes or until your desired level of doneness. Use a spoon to carefully lift the eggs from the water. Allow them to rest on a paper towel-lined plate to remove excess moisture.

3. In a non-stick pan over medium heat, add the kale and water. Use a lid to steam for 2 to 3 minutes until the liquid evaporates, and the kale becomes tender.

4. Serve the quinoa in bowls, add the kale and poached eggs on top, season with a pinch of salt, and enjoy!

NUTRITION - AMOUNT PER SERVING

Calories	313	Sugar	1g
Fat	12g	Protein	19g
Carbs	30g	Cholesterol	372mg
Fiber	4g	Sodium	451mg

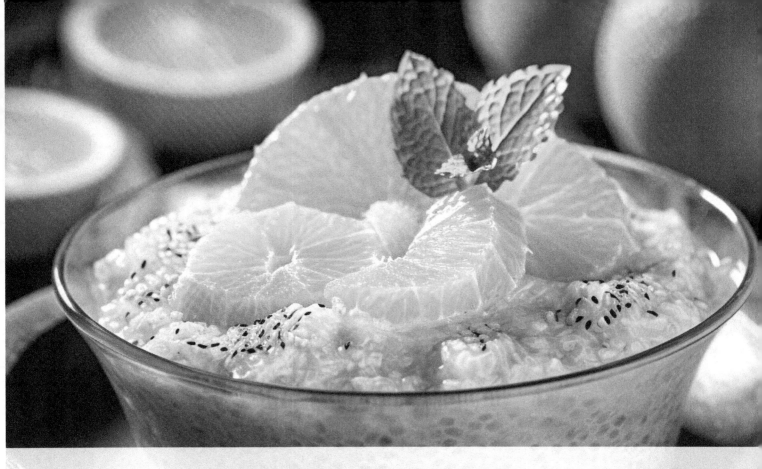

Orange Creamsicle Chia Pudding

 4 Hours 10 Minutes

 1 Serving

INGREDIENTS

- ½ cup Canned Coconut Milk
- 2 tbsps Orange Juice
- ¾ tsp Maple Syrup
- ⅛ tsp Vanilla Extract
- 1 ¾ tbsps Chia Seeds
- ⅛ Navel Orange (peeled and diced)

INSTRUCTIONS

1. In a resealable container, whisk together coconut milk, orange juice, maple syrup, and vanilla extract. Whisk in chia seeds.

2. Cover with an airtight lid and refrigerate for four hours or overnight to set. In the morning, divide into bowls and top with diced oranges.

NUTRITION - AMOUNT PER SERVING

Calories	322	Sugar	9g
Fat	25g	Protein	5g
Carbs	20g	Cholesterol	0mg
Fiber	7g	Sodium	31mg

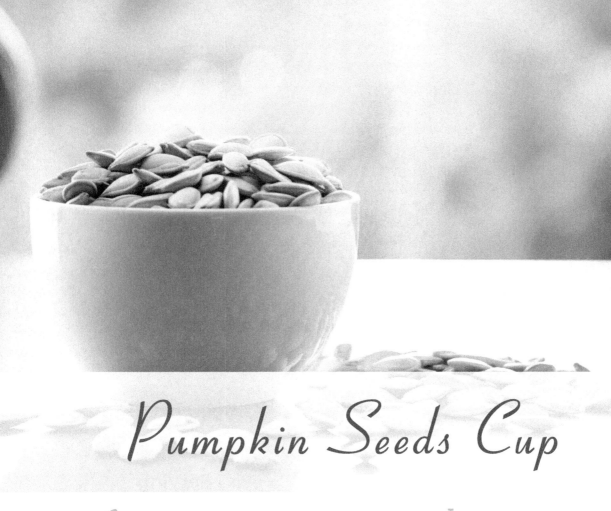

Pumpkin Seeds Cup

 1 Minute

 1 Serving

INGREDIENTS

- 1/4 cup Pumpkin Seeds

INSTRUCTIONS

1. Place in a bowl and enjoy!

NUTRITION - AMOUNT PER SERVING

Calories	180	Sugar	10g
Fat	16g	Protein	10g
Carbs	3g	Cholesterol	0mg
Fiber	2g	Sodium	2mg

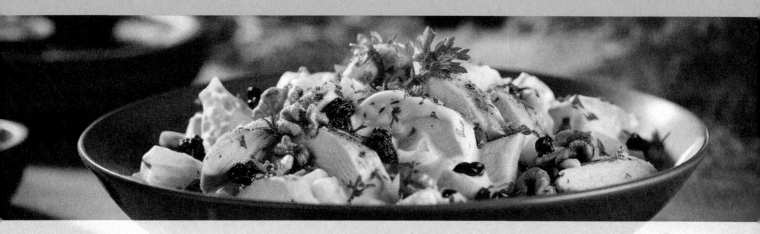

Creamy Dill Salad with Chicken

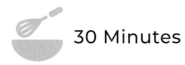 **30 Minutes**

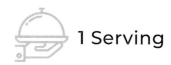 **1 Serving**

INGREDIENTS

- 113 grams Chicken Breast
- Sea Salt & Black Pepper (to taste)
- 1 1/2 tsps Extra Virgin Olive Oil
- 3/4 tsp Apple Cider Vinegar
- 1 1/2 tsps Water
- 2 2/3 tbsps Fresh Dill (chopped, divided)
- 1/4 cup Walnuts (divided)
- 1/2 head Romaine Hearts (chopped)
- 1/4 cup Black Olives

INSTRUCTIONS

1. Preheat oven to 400°F (205°C). Lay the chicken breast(s) on a baking sheet and season with salt and pepper. Roast them in the oven for about half an hour.

2. As the chicken is baking, prepare your salad dressing. In a blender, blend together the oil, apple cider vinegar, water, a quarter of the dill, and a quarter of the walnuts until you achieve a smooth, creamy consistency. If needed, add a bit more water to reach your desired thickness. Season with salt to taste and set the dressing aside.

3. In a spacious bowl, toss together the romaine, the rest of the dill, the remaining walnuts, and black olives. Add the creamy dressing to the salad and thoroughly combine until everything is evenly coated.

4. Place salad in a bowl and top with sliced chicken.

NUTRITION - AMOUNT PER SERVING

Calories	434	Sugar	1g
Fat	33g	Protein	31g
Carbs	7g	Cholesterol	82mg
Fiber	3g	Sodium	301mg

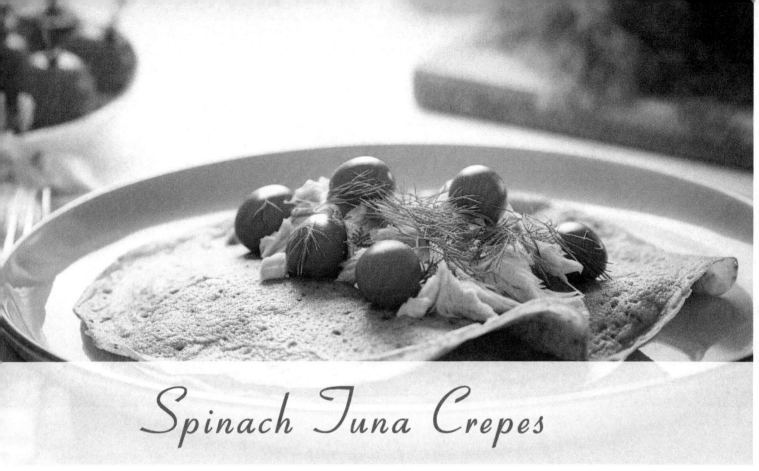

Spinach Tuna Crepes

 35 Minutes

 2 Servings

INGREDIENTS

- 1 cup Baby Spinach
- 2 tbsps Parsley
- 1 cup Unsweetened Almond Milk
- 1 Egg
- 2/3 cup Brown Rice Flour
- Sea Salt & Black Pepper (to taste)
- 1 tbsp Extra Virgin Olive Oil
- 1 can Tuna (drained and flaked)
- 3/4 cup Cherry Tomatoes (halved)
- 1 1/2 tsps Fresh Dill (chopped)

INSTRUCTIONS

1. Blend the spinach, parsley, almond milk, and eggs until smooth. Slowly add the flour until thoroughly combined. Season with salt and pepper to taste.

2. Brush a medium skillet with olive oil over medium heat. As soon as it's hot, pour ¼ cup of the batter into it, then gently spread the batter to form a thin crepe by swirling the skillet gently. Cook for approximately 1 to 2 minutes. Flip and cook for another 30 seconds. Repeat with the remaining batter.

3. Divide crepes onto plates. Spoon tuna in the middle along with cherry tomatoes. Sprinkle dill on top. Roll the crepes and enjoy.

NUTRITION - AMOUNT PER SERVING

Calories	387	Sugar	2g
Fat	13g	Protein	25g
Carbs	44g	Cholesterol	123mg
Fiber	4g	Sodium	341mg

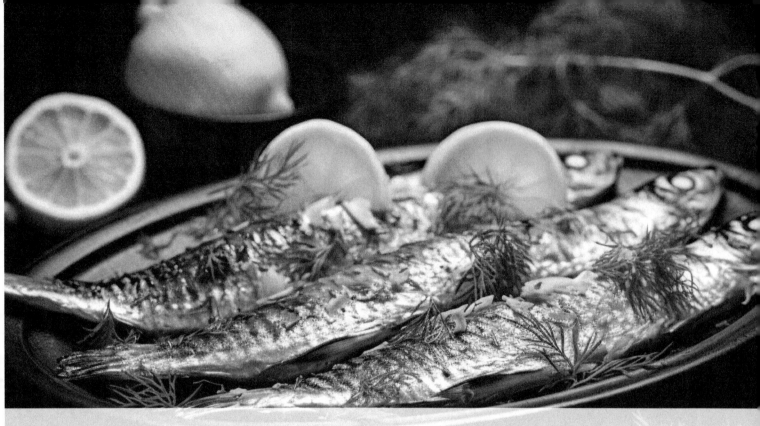

Broiled Mackerel

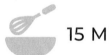 15 Minutes

 1 Serving

INGREDIENTS

- 113 grams Mackerel Fillet (patted dry)
- ¾ tsp Extra Virgin Olive Oil
- ⅛ tsp Sea Salt

INSTRUCTIONS

1. Set your oven to broil and move the rack to the top rung.

2. Place mackerel fillets on a baking sheet and coat in oil. Season with salt and broil for 6 to 7 minutes. Cooking times may vary due to thickness. If more time is needed, lower the heat to 350°F (177°C) and cook until the flesh is opaque in the centre.

3. Place on a serving dish and enjoy!

NUTRITION - AMOUNT PER SERVING

Calories	262	Sugar	0g
Fat	19g	Protein	21g
Carbs	0g	Cholesterol	79mg
Fiber	0g	Sodium	397mg

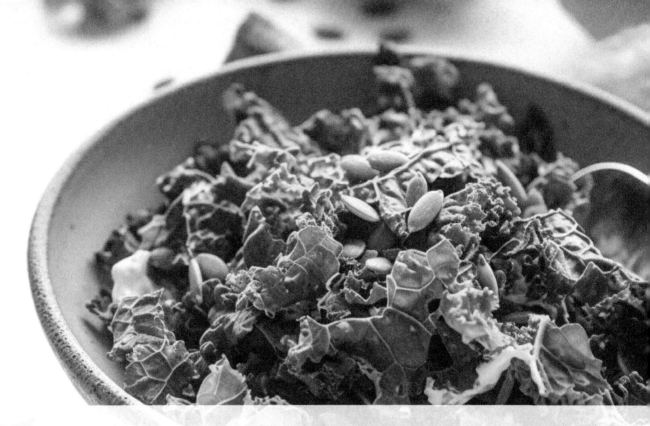

Curried Kale Salad

 15 Minutes

 2 Servings

INGREDIENTS

- 1/4 cup Lemon Juice
- 2 tbsps Tahini
- 1 tbsp Coconut Aminos
- 1 tsp Maple Syrup
- 1 1/2 tsps Curry Powder
- 1/8 tsp Sea Salt
- 75 grams Kale Leaves (washed, dried, thinly sliced)
- 2 tbsps Pumpkin Seeds

INSTRUCTIONS

1. In a small bowl, whisk together the lemon juice, tahini, coconut aminos, maple syrup, curry powder and sea salt to make the dressing.

2. Add the kale leaves to a large bowl and add the dressing. Massage the dressing into the kale leaves using your hands. Garnish with pumpkin seeds.

NUTRITION - AMOUNT PER SERVING

Calories	175	Sugar	5g
Fat	13g	Protein	6g
Carbs	12g	Cholesterol	0mg
Fiber	4g	Sodium	322mg

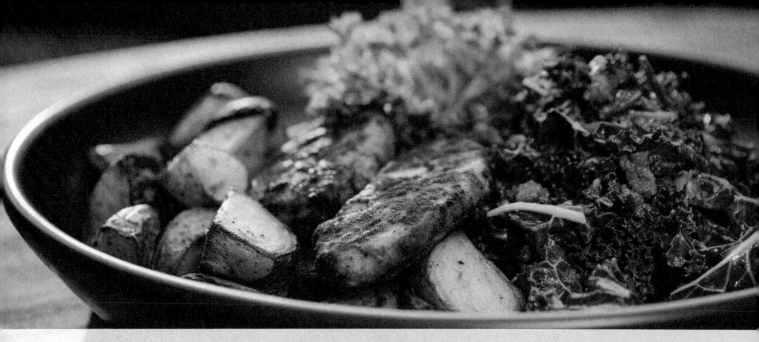

Cajun Chicken, Potatoes & Kale

 35 Minutes

 2 Servings

INGREDIENTS

- 1 Yellow Potato (medium, diced into 1/2 inch thick pieces)
- 1 1/2 tsps Extra Virgin Olive Oil
- 1 tbsp Cajun Spice (divided)
- 1 1/2 tsps Coconut Oil (divided)
- 227 grams Extra Lean Ground Chicken
- 75 grams Kale Leaves (sliced)
- Sea Salt & Black Pepper (to taste)

INSTRUCTIONS

1. Preheat the oven to 430°F (222°C). Line a baking sheet with parchment paper.

2. In a bowl, toss the diced potatoes with olive oil and half of the cajun spice. Ensure they are well coated. Spread the coated diced potatoes on the baking sheet and bake for 30 minutes. Toss them at the halfway mark.

3. While the potatoes are baking, heat half the coconut oil in a skillet over medium heat. Add the ground chicken and sauté for about 10 minutes, ensuring it's thoroughly cooked, and break it up as it cooks. Add the remaining Cajun spice and continue sautéing until the spice is evenly distributed. Transfer the cooked ground chicken to a bowl and cover it to keep it warm.

4. Place the skillet back over medium heat and add the remaining coconut oil. Add in the kale, season with sea salt and black pepper then sauté just until wilted. Turn off the heat.

5. Divide cajun chicken, potatoes and sauteed kale between plates.

NUTRITION - AMOUNT PER SERVING

Calories	317	Sugar	1g
Fat	17g	Protein	23g
Carbs	20g	Cholesterol	98mg
Fiber	4g	Sodium	424mg

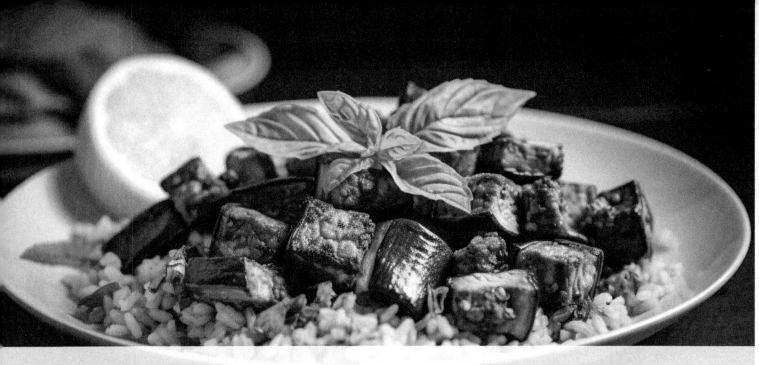

Grilled Tempeh & Eggplant with Rice

 50 Minutes

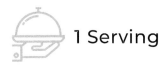 1 Serving

INGREDIENTS

- 1/4 cup Brown Rice (dry)
- 2/3 tsp Sesame Oil
- 2 tsps Tamari
- 1 tsp Maple Syrup
- 1 tsp Apple Cider Vinegar
- 1/3 Eggplant (small, peeled, seeds removed, sliced)
- 113 grams Tempeh (sliced)
- 1 cup Baby Spinach
- 1 1/3 tbsps Lemon Juice (to taste)

INSTRUCTIONS

1. Cook the brown rice according to package directions and set aside.

2. In a baking dish, combine the sesame oil, tamari, maple syrup, and apple cider vinegar. Add the eggplant and tempeh, brushing all sides with the marinade. Let sit for 5 to 10 minutes.

3. Grill the eggplant over medium heat for 10 minutes on one side, and 6 to 8 minutes on the other side, or until fork tender. Grill the tempeh for 8 minutes, flipping halfway. Brush on any leftover marinade as needed.

4. Place the brown rice, spinach, eggplant, and tempeh on a plate. Drizzle lemon juice and enjoy!

NUTRITION - AMOUNT PER SERVING

Calories	496	Sugar	12g
Fat	17g	Protein	30g
Carbs	62g	Cholesterol	0mg
Fiber	8g	Sodium	711mg

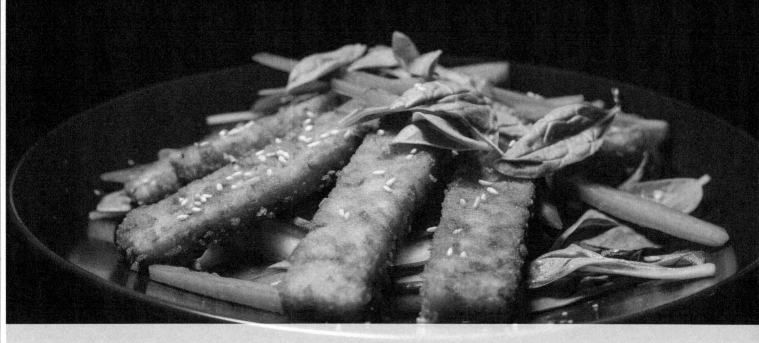

Pan Fried Tofu Spinach Salad

 20 Minutes

 2 Servings

INGREDIENTS

- 2 tbsps Avocado Oil (divided)
- 200 grams Tofu (extra-firm, cut into thin strips)
- 1 1/2 tbsps Tamari (divided)
- 1 1/2 tsps Maple Syrup
- 1 1/2 tsps Lime Juice
- 1 cup Baby Spinach
- 1/2 Cucumber (medium, cut into matchsticks)
- 1 Carrot (medium, peeled and cut into matchsticks)

INSTRUCTIONS

1. Heat half of the oil in a non-stick pan over medium heat. Add the tofu strips and cook for 5 to 6 minutes per side until browned. To avoid overcrowding, cook in batches. Reduce the heat to low and remove the pan from the heat. Add ⅔ of the tamari and gently swirl the pan to coat the tofu. Place the pan back on the burner and cook for about 1 to 2 minutes per side. When crispy, transfer to a plate lined with paper towels.

2. In a bowl mix the maple syrup, lime juice, the remaining oil, and tamari.

3. To serve, divide the spinach between bowls. Top with the cucumber, carrot, and tofu. Drizzle with the dressing and enjoy!

NUTRITION - AMOUNT PER SERVING

Calories	256	Sugar	7g
Fat	19g	Protein	13g
Carbs	12g	Cholesterol	0mg
Fiber	3g	Sodium	793mg

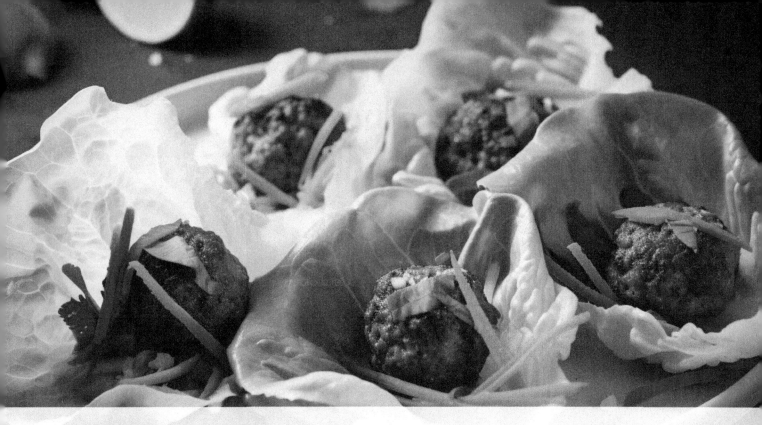

Meatball Lettuce Wraps

 40 Minutes

 2 Servings

INGREDIENTS

- 213 grams Extra Lean Ground Beef
- Sea Salt & Black Pepper (to taste)
- ¾ cup Grated Carrot
- ¼ cup Parsley
- 1 head Boston Lettuce (peeled apart into leaves and washed)
- ½ Lime (cut into wedges)

INSTRUCTIONS

1. Preheat the oven to 400°F (205°C) and line a baking sheet with parchment paper.

2. In a large bowl mix together the ground beef, salt, and pepper. Roll the beef into roughly one-inch balls and place them on the baking sheet. Bake in the oven for 20 to 25 minutes or until cooked through.

3. Divide the cooked meatballs, carrot, and parsley between lettuce leaves. Squeeze lime juice on top and enjoy!

NUTRITION - AMOUNT PER SERVING

Calories	210	Sugar	2g
Fat	11g	Protein	22g
Carbs	5g	Cholesterol	69mg
Fiber	2g	Sodium	103mg

Dinners

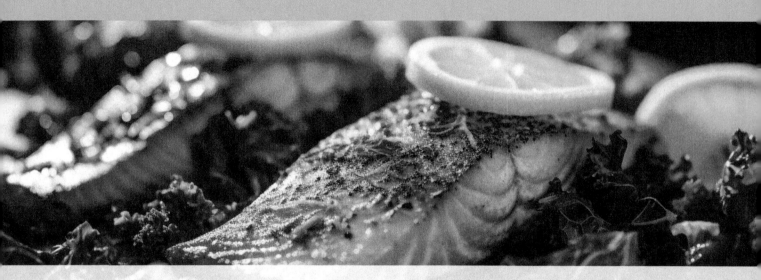

Massaged Kale Salad with Salmon

 20 Minutes

 1 Serving

INGREDIENTS

- 75 grams Kale Leaves (chopped)
- 1/2 Lemon (juiced)
- 1 tbsp Hemp Seeds
- Sea Salt & Black Pepper (to taste)
- 2 tbsps Extra Virgin Olive Oil (divided)
- 160 grams Salmon Fillet

INSTRUCTIONS

1. Add the kale leaves to a bowl with the lemon juice, hemp seeds, salt and pepper, and half the olive oil. Massage the dressing into the kale with your hands for 2 to 3 minutes, until the kale is softened. Set it aside.

2. Heat a skillet over medium heat and brush with the remaining olive oil. Season the salmon with salt and pepper. Place the salmon in the pan skin-side down, cooking for about 3 minutes. Then turn over and cook for another 1 to 2 minutes, until the flesh is completely opaque throughout.

3. Plate the massaged kale and top with the salmon, adding an extra squeeze of lemon.

NUTRITION - AMOUNT PER SERVING

Calories	535	Sugar	1g
Fat	41g	Protein	41g
Carbs	6g	Cholesterol	82mg
Fiber	4g	Sodium	166mg

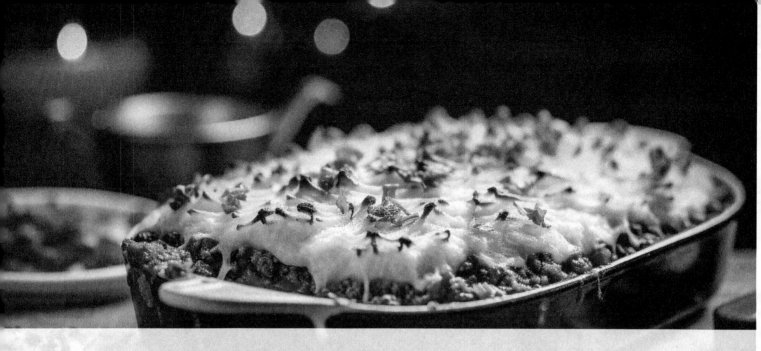

Potato Shepherd's Pie

 35 Minutes

 2 Servings

INGREDIENTS

- 1 Yellow Potato (large, peeled and roughly chopped)
- 1 1/2 tsps Extra Virgin Olive Oil (divided)
- 1/2 tsp Sea Salt (divided)
- 227 grams Extra Lean Ground Beef
- 1/2 Carrot (medium, finely chopped)
- 1 1/2 tsps Italian Seasoning
- 1/2 tsp Black Pepper

INSTRUCTIONS

1. Put the potatoes in a medium pot with sufficient water to cover them. Bring it to a boil and cook until the potatoes are tender, about 10 minutes. Drain the potatoes and then mash them with the oil and half of the salt. Set them aside.

2. In a skillet over medium-high heat, combine the beef, carrot, Italian seasoning, black pepper, and the rest of the salt. Sauté for 6 to 8 minutes until the beef is thoroughly browned and the veggies have softened. Drain any excess liquid.

3. Set oven broiler to high or 550°F (290°C).

4. Spread the beef filling in a baking dish. Spoon the mashed potatoes on top evenly. Brush the top with the remaining oil and place it under the broiler for 10 to 15 minutes, or until browned. Divide onto serving plates and enjoy!

NUTRITION - AMOUNT PER SERVING

Calories	320	Sugar	2g
Fat	15g	Protein	25g
Carbs	21g	Cholesterol	74mg
Fiber	3g	Sodium	682mg

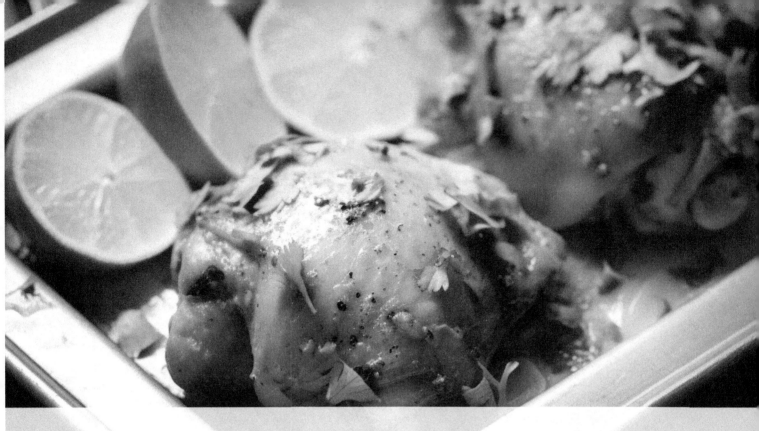

Baked Cilantro Lime Chicken

 1 Hour 30 Minutes 1 Serving

INGREDIENTS

- 113 grams Chicken Thighs (boneless, skinless)
- 2 tbsps Cilantro (finely chopped)
- 1/2 Lime (juiced, divided)
- 1 1/2 tsps Avocado Oil
- 1/8 tsp Sea Salt

INSTRUCTIONS

1. Add the chicken thighs, cilantro, half of the lime juice, avocado oil, and sea salt to a zipper-lock bag or shallow bowl. Once the chicken is coated in the marinade, let it sit in the fridge for at least an hour. For maximum flavor, marinate overnight.

2. Preheat the oven to 400°F (204°C) and remove the chicken thighs from the marinade. Using a paper towel, pat dry before placing the chicken thighs in a baking dish.

3. Bake the chicken for 20 to 25 minutes. Once the thighs are thoroughly cooked, remove them from the oven and drizzle with the remaining lime juice. Season with additional salt if needed. Rest the chicken for approximately 5 minutes before serving.

NUTRITION - AMOUNT PER SERVING

Calories	205	Sugar	0g
Fat	12g	Protein	22g
Carbs	2g	Cholesterol	107mg
Fiber	0g	Sodium	404mg

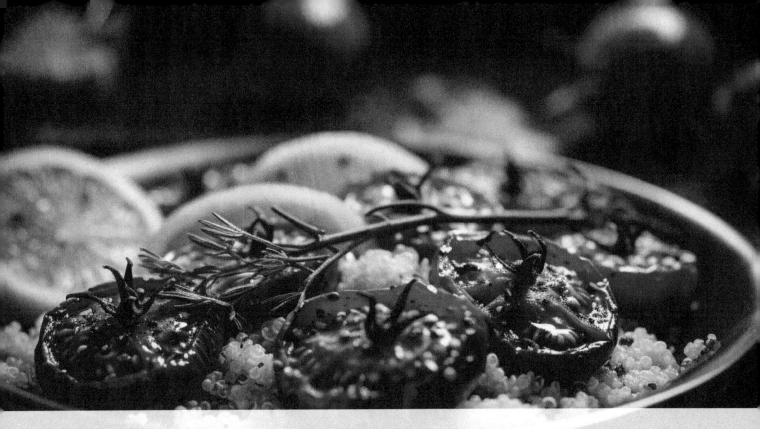

Tomato & Thyme Quinoa

 30 Minutes

 1 Serving

INGREDIENTS

- ⅓ cup Cherry Tomatoes (cut in half)
- 2 ¼ tsps Extra Virgin Olive Oil (divided)
- 1/16 tsp Sea Salt
- ¼ cup Quinoa (uncooked)
- ½ cup Water
- ¾ tsp Thyme (chopped)
- 1 ⅛ tsps Lemon Juice

INSTRUCTIONS

1. Preheat the oven to 400°F (204°C) and line a baking sheet with parchment paper. Place the tomatoes cut side up. Drizzle with half the extra virgin olive oil and sea salt and cook for 10 minutes. Remove, flip the tomatoes and place back in the oven for 12 to 15 minutes.

2. Meanwhile, combine quinoa and water together in a saucepan. Place over high heat and bring to a boil. Once boiling, reduce heat to a simmer and cover with a lid. Let it simmer for 13 to 15 minutes or until the water is absorbed.

3. Add the quinoa to a large bowl along with the tomatoes and thyme. Add the remaining extra virgin olive oil and lemon juice. Toss to combine. Serve and enjoy!

NUTRITION - AMOUNT PER SERVING

Calories	258	Sugar	2g
Fat	13g	Protein	7g
Carbs	30g	Cholesterol	0mg
Fiber	4g	Sodium	81mg

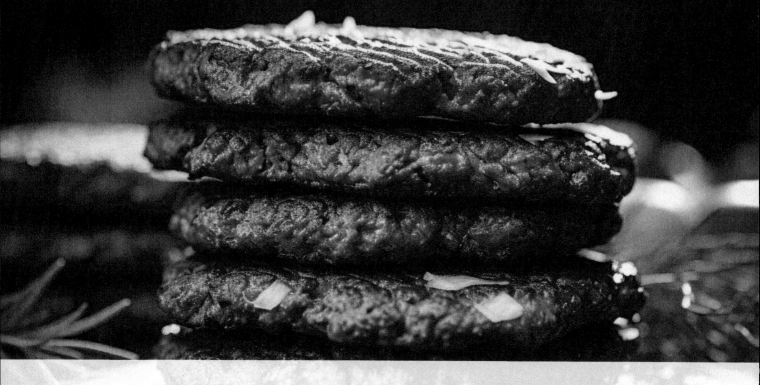

Maple Beef Burgers

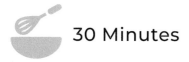 30 Minutes

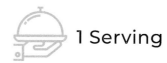 1 Serving

INGREDIENTS

- 113 grams Extra Lean Ground Beef
- 1½ tsps Maple Syrup
- ¼ tsp Dried Thyme
- ½ tsp Ground Sage
- ¼ tsp Sea Salt
- 1 ½ tsps Coconut Oil

INSTRUCTIONS

1. In a bowl, mix the ground beef, maple syrup, thyme, sage, and salt.

2. Divide the mixture and shape it into half-inch thick patties. Put the patties on a parchment paper lined tray and chill in the freezer for about 15 minutes.

3. In a large pan, heat the coconut oil over medium heat. Fry each burger patty until cooked through, about 4 to 6 minutes per side.

4. Set aside to cool slightly.

NUTRITION - AMOUNT PER SERVING

Calories	287	Sugar	6g
Fat	18g	Protein	23g
Carbs	7g	Cholesterol	73mg
Fiber	0g	Sodium	666mg

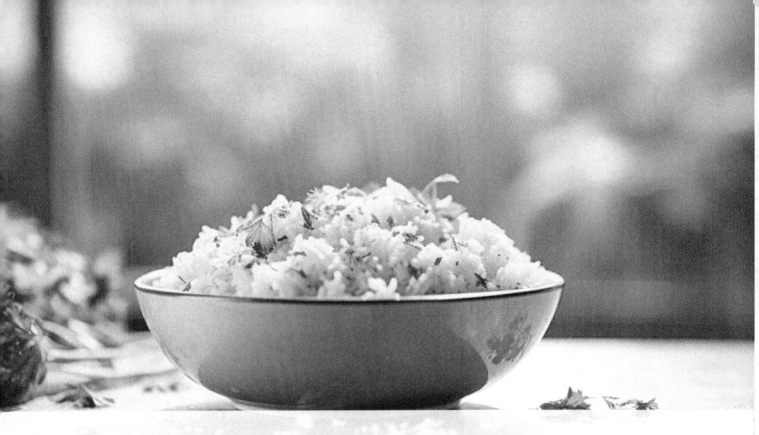

Herbed Rice

 25 Minutes

 1 Serving

INGREDIENTS

- 3/4 cup Vegetable Broth (low sodium)
- 1/3 cup Basmati Rice (uncooked)
- 1 1/2 tsps Butter
- 2 tbsps Parsley (chopped)
- 2 tbsps Fresh Dill (chopped)
- Sea Salt & Black Pepper (to taste)

INSTRUCTIONS

1. Add the broth and rice to a pot and bring to a boil. Lower the heat and simmer for 15 minutes.

2. Remove from heat and stir in the butter, parsley, dill, salt and pepper. Cover and let rest for 10 minutes.

NUTRITION - AMOUNT PER SERVING

Calories	331	Sugar	2g
Fat	6g	Protein	6g
Carbs	62g	Cholesterol	15mg
Fiber	2g	Sodium	89mg

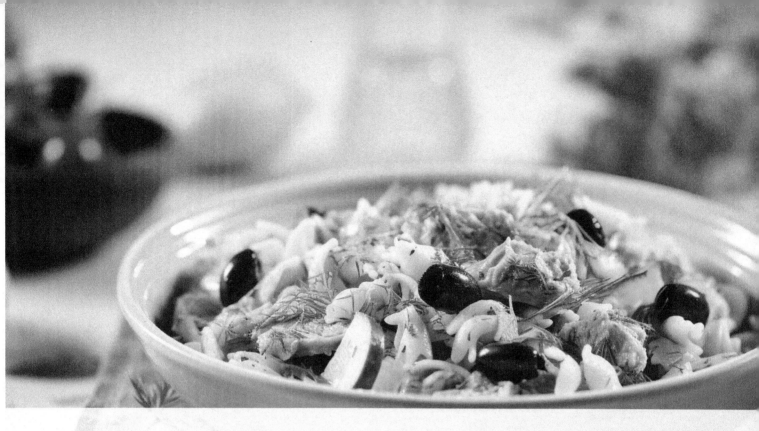

Zucchini & Tuna Pasta Salad

 15 Minutes

 2 Servings

INGREDIENTS

- ½ cup Brown Rice Macaroni (dry)
- 65 grams Zucchini (small, diced)
- ¼ cup Black Olives (pitted, chopped)
- ½ tsp Oregano (dried)
- 1 can Tuna (drained, crumbled)
- 1 tbsp Extra Virgin Olive Oil

INSTRUCTIONS

1. Cook the macaroni following the instructions on the package. Drain, rinse, and set aside to cool.

2. Combine all the ingredients including the cooled pasta in a serving bowl and mix to coat.

3. Divide evenly between bowls and enjoy!

NUTRITION - AMOUNT PER SERVING

Calories	263	Sugar	1g
Fat	10g	Protein	19g
Carbs	24g	Cholesterol	30mg
Fiber	2g	Sodium	327mg

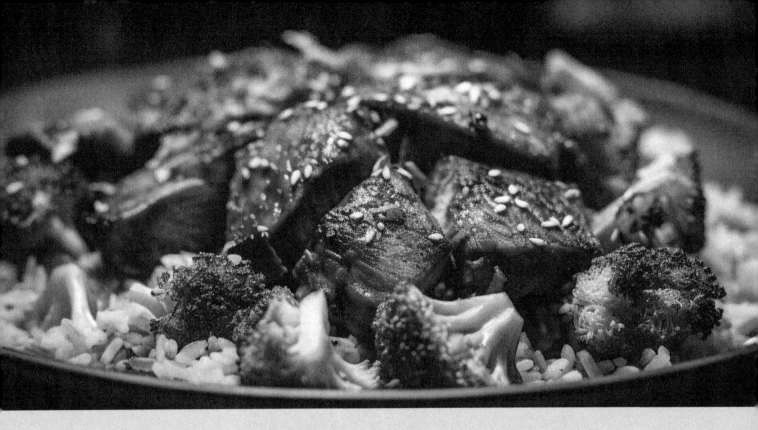

Cumin Roasted Chicken & Broccoli

 30 Minutes

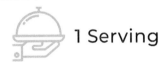 1 Serving

INGREDIENTS

- 1/4 cup Brown Basmati Rice (uncooked)
- 2 1/4 tsps Cumin Seeds
- 3/4 tsp Fennel Seeds
- 1/4 tsp Sea Salt
- 75 grams Broccoli Florets (chopped)
- 1 1/8 tsps Coconut Oil (melted, divided)
- 150 grams Chicken Breast (cut into one-inch cubes)

INSTRUCTIONS

1. Cook the basmati rice according to the packaging. Preheat oven to 350°F (175°C). Line a baking sheet with parchment paper.

2. While your rice is cooking, coarsely grind the cumin and fennel seeds using a spice grinder or a mortar and pestle. Then, add salt to the mixture and set it aside.

3. In a bowl, toss the broccoli with half of the coconut oil and half of the spices. Then, transfer the coated broccoli to one side of the baking sheet.

4. In the same bowl, coat the chicken with the remaining coconut oil and spices. Transfer the chicken breast cubes to the baking sheet and bake for 20 minutes or until cooked through.

5. Place the rice, chicken, and broccoli on a plate and enjoy!

NUTRITION - AMOUNT PER SERVING

Calories	434	Sugar	1g
Fat	12g	Protein	40g
Carbs	43g	Cholesterol	110mg
Fiber	4g	Sodium	692mg

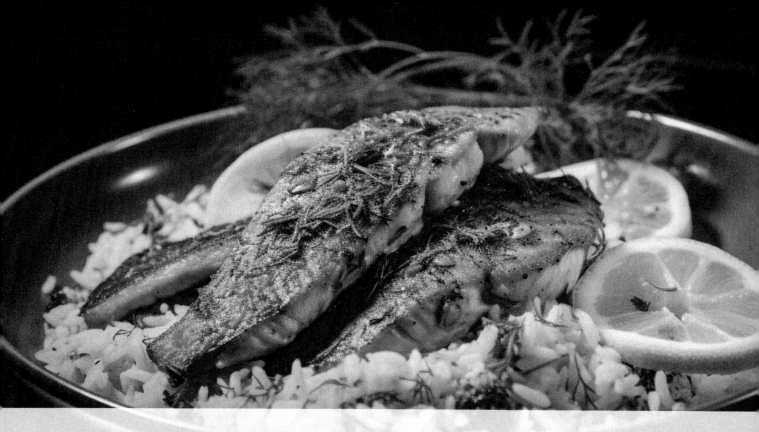

Pan-Fried Trout with Herbed Rice

 30 Minutes

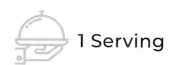 1 Serving

INGREDIENTS

- ¾ cup Vegetable Broth (low sodium)
- ⅓ cup Basmati Rice (uncooked)
- 1 tbsp Butter (divided)
- 2 tbsps Parsley (chopped)
- 2 tbsps Fresh Dill (chopped)
- Sea Salt & Black Pepper (to taste)
- 1 Rainbow Trout Fillet (patted dry)

INSTRUCTIONS

1. Add the broth and rice to a pot and bring to a boil. Lower the heat and simmer for 15 minutes. Remove from heat and stir in half the butter, parsley, dill, salt and pepper. Cover and let rest for 10 minutes.

2. Season the trout with salt and pepper.

3. Melt the remaining butter in a skillet over medium-high heat. Cook the trout for 3 to 5 minutes, flipping halfway, or until browned and cooked through.

4. Serve the herbed rice and trout on a plate and enjoy!

NUTRITION - AMOUNT PER SERVING

Calories	571	Sugar	2g
Fat	17g	Protein	39g
Carbs	62g	Cholesterol	124mg
Fiber	2g	Sodium	139mg

Snacks

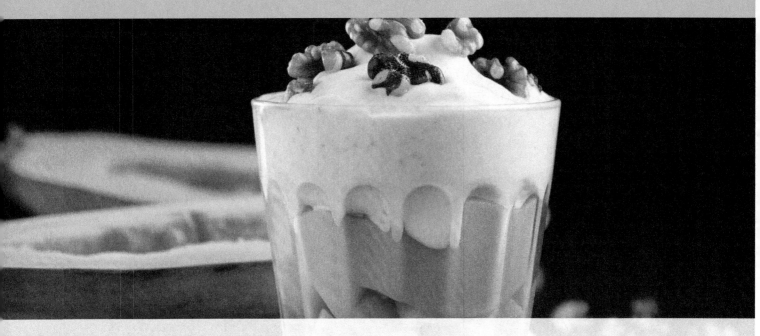

Papaya with Yogurt & Walnuts

 5 Minutes

 1 Serving

INGREDIENTS

- 1 cup Papaya
  (peeled, seeds removed, chopped)
- 1/8 tsp Cinnamon (to taste)
- 1/2 cup Coconut Yogurt
  (unsweetened)
- 1/4 cup Walnuts

INSTRUCTIONS

1. Place the papaya into a cup and top with cinnamon, yogurt and walnuts.

NUTRITION - AMOUNT PER SERVING

Calories	312	Sugar	12g
Fat	23g	Protein	6g
Carbs	26g	Cholesterol	0mg
Fiber	6g	Sodium	37mg

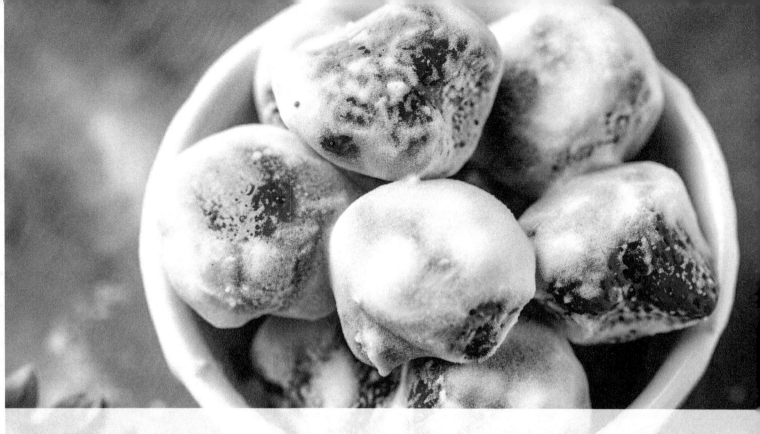

Frozen Coconut Yogurt Covered Strawberries

 40 Minutes

 1 Serving

INGREDIENTS

- ½ cup Unsweetened Coconut Yogurt
- 65 grams Strawberries

INSTRUCTIONS

1. Line a baking sheet with parchment paper.
2. Add the yogurt to a bowl followed by the strawberries. Coat each strawberry in yogurt. Work in batches if needed.
3. Spread the yogurt covered strawberries out in an even layer on the baking sheet. Freeze for 25 to 30 minutes.

NUTRITION - AMOUNT PER SERVING

Calories	76	Sugar	4g
Fat	4g	Protein	1g
Carbs	11g	Cholesterol	0mg
Fiber	3g	Sodium	25mg

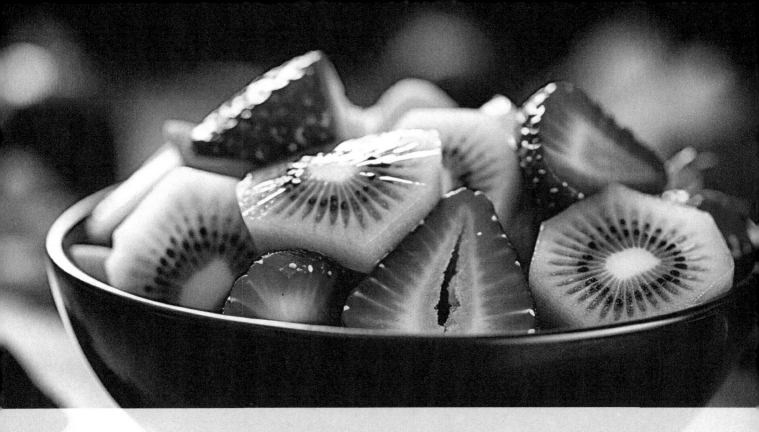

Kiwi & Strawberries

 5 Minutes

 2 Servings

INGREDIENTS

- 1 Kiwi (sliced)
- 55 grams Strawberries

INSTRUCTIONS

1. Serve the kiwi with the strawberries.

NUTRITION - AMOUNT PER SERVING

Calories	30	Sugar	4g
Fat	0g	Protein	1g
Carbs	7g	Cholesterol	0mg
Fiber	2g	Sodium	1mg

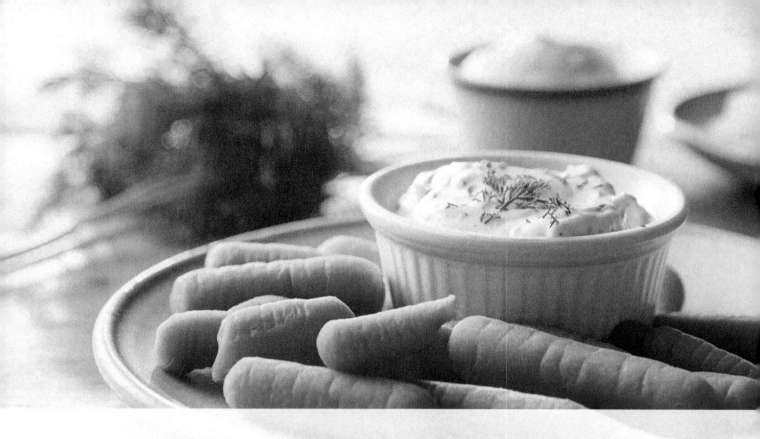

Lemon Dill Yogurt Dip & Carrots

 5 Minutes

 3 Servings

INGREDIENTS

- ¾ cup Unsweetened Coconut Yogurt
- ¾ Lemon (juiced)
- 3 tbsps Fresh Dill (finely chopped)
- 1 ½ cups Baby Carrots

INSTRUCTIONS

1. Combine the yogurt, lemon juice, and dill in a bowl.
2. Serve with the baby carrots.

NUTRITION - AMOUNT PER SERVING

Calories	60	Sugar	5g
Fat	2g	Protein	0g
Carbs	11g	Cholesterol	0mg
Fiber	3g	Sodium	77mg

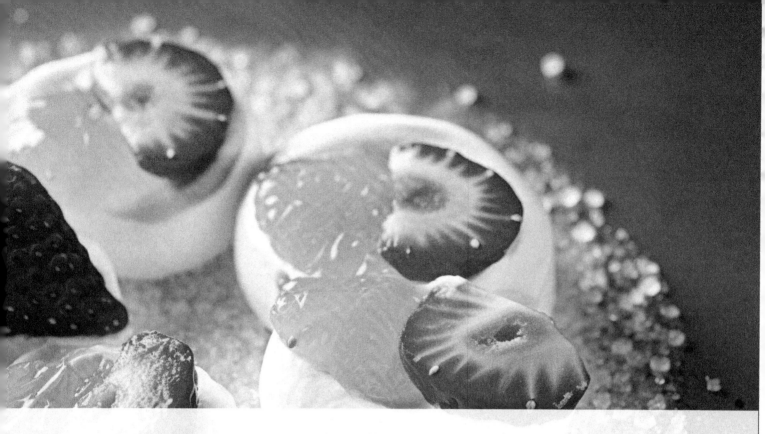

Orange & Strawberry Frozen Yogurt Bites

 2 Hours 10 Minutes   3 Servings

INGREDIENTS

- 2/3 cup Unsweetened Coconut Yogurt
- 1 3/4 tsps Maple Syrup
- 2/3 tsp Vanilla Extract
- 1 1/4 Navel Orange (small, peeled and sectioned)
- 3 1/4 tbsps Strawberries

INSTRUCTIONS

1. Line a baking sheet with parchment paper or a non-stick baking mat. Combine the yogurt, maple syrup, and vanilla in a bowl.

2. Drop one heaping tablespoon of yogurt onto the baking sheet. Continue until all of the yogurt is evenly divided onto the baking sheet. Divide the oranges and strawberries evenly among the yogurt.

3. Freeze for two to three hours or until frozen.

NUTRITION - AMOUNT PER SERVING

Calories	65	Sugar	8g
Fat	2g	Protein	1g
Carbs	13g	Cholesterol	0mg
Fiber	2g	Sodium	11mg

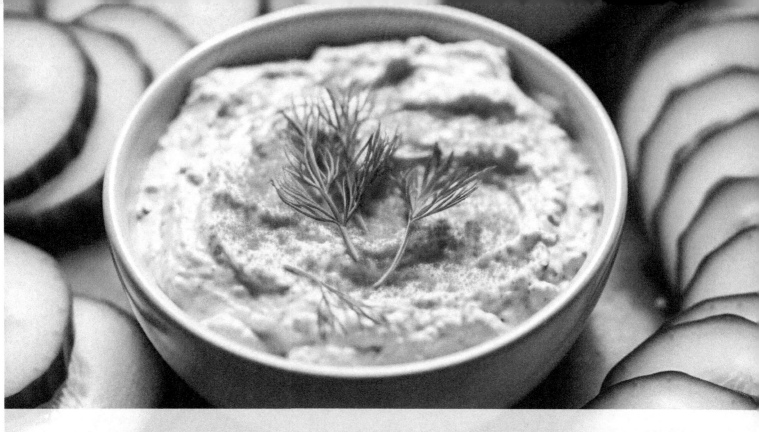

Cucumbers & Salmon Dip

 5 Minutes

 1 Serving

INGREDIENTS

- 107 grams Canned Wild Salmon (drained)
- 2 tbsps Unsweetened Coconut Yogurt
- 1 ½ tsps Fresh Dill (chopped)
- 1/16 tsp Sea Salt
- ½ Cucumber (large, sliced)

INSTRUCTIONS

1. Combine the salmon, yogurt, dill, and salt in a food processor and blend until smooth.

2. Serve the salmon dip with the cucumber slices.

NUTRITION - AMOUNT PER SERVING

Calories	205	Sugar	3g
Fat	7g	Protein	29g
Carbs	7g	Cholesterol	70mg
Fiber	1g	Sodium	568mg

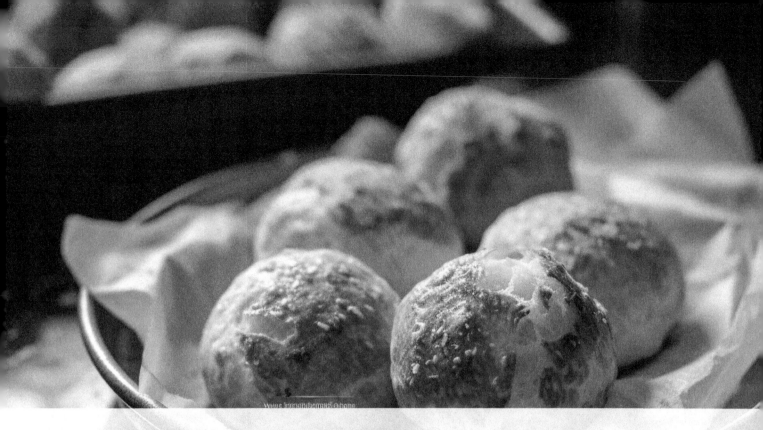

Brazilian Cheese Bread

 40 Minutes

 1 Serving

INGREDIENTS

- 2 tbsps Unsweetened Almond Milk
- 1 tbsp Extra Virgin Olive Oil
- 1/8 tsp Sea Salt
- 1/4 cup Tapioca Flour
- 1/4 Egg
- 2 2/3 tbsps Parmigiano Reggiano (shredded)

INSTRUCTIONS

1. Preheat the oven to 350°F (175°C) and line a baking sheet with parchment paper.

2. Place the milk, oil, and salt in a medium saucepan. Then, over medium heat, bring to a gentle boil, stirring occasionally. Before removing from the heat, simmer for 1 minute.

3. Add the tapioca flour and milk mixture to a bowl of a stand mixer. Beat until it is smooth and cool for a few minutes at medium speed with a paddle attachment.

4. Add the egg and beat it until fully incorporated. Add the cheese and continue beating until a very sticky dough forms. Using an ice cream scoop, place the dough onto the baking sheet, spacing the cheese balls two inches apart.

5. Bake for 22 to 25 minutes or until they have puffed and are golden brown.

NUTRITION - AMOUNT PER SERVING

Calories	314	Sugar	0g
Fat	20g	Protein	8g
Carbs	26g	Cholesterol	63mg
Fiber	0g	Sodium	453mg

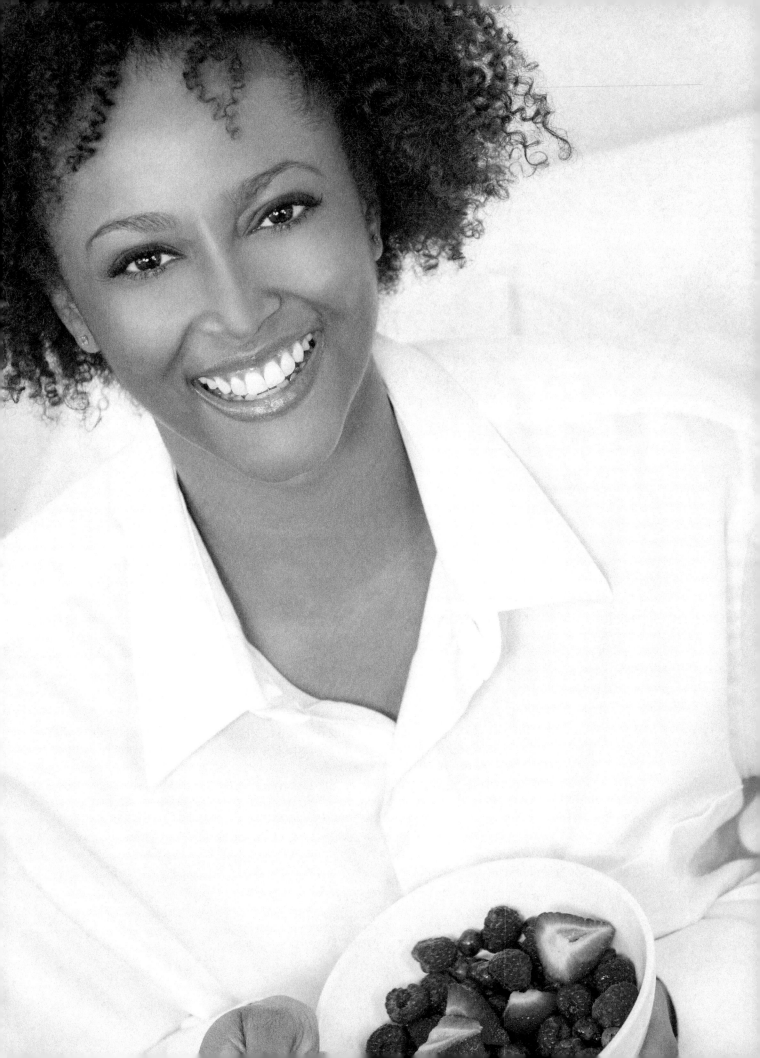

BONUS RECIPES

Desserts

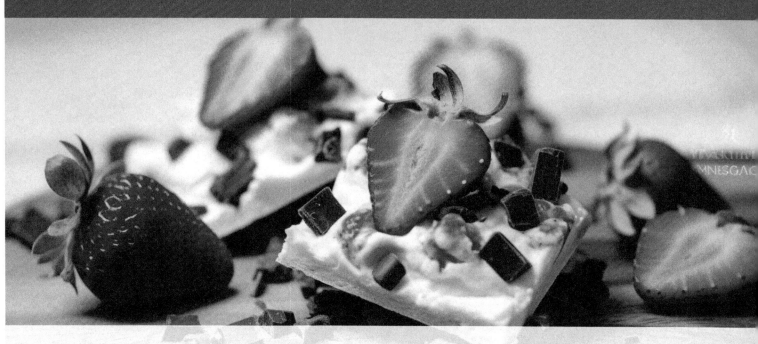

Chocolate & Strawberry Yogurt Bark

 8 Hours

 5 Servings

INGREDIENTS

- 1 cup Unsweetened Coconut Yogurt
- 1 1/2 tsps Maple Syrup
- 1/4 tsp Vanilla Extract
- 1/4 cup Strawberries (sliced)
- 11 grams Dark Chocolate (chopped)

INSTRUCTIONS

1. Line a baking sheet with parchment paper.

2. Stir the yogurt, maple syrup, and vanilla extract together in a bowl. Pour the mixture onto the baking sheet and evenly spread it out.

3. Top with the strawberries and dark chocolate. Set in the freezer overnight. Break apart and enjoy!

NUTRITION - AMOUNT PER SERVING

Calories	43	Sugar	2g
Fat	2g	Protein	0g
Carbs	5g	Cholesterol	0mg
Fiber	1g	Sodium	11mg

192

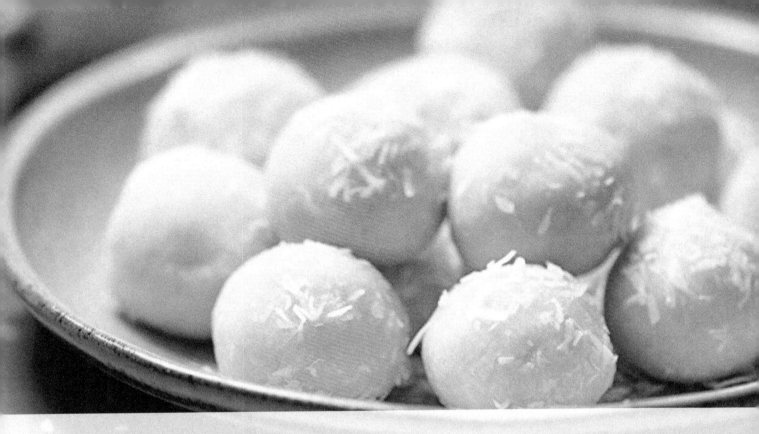

Lemon Coconut Power Balls

 1 Hour 15 Minutes

 5 Servings

INGREDIENTS

- 1/2 cup Unsweetened Shredded Coconut
- 1/4 cup Coconut Butter
- 2 1/2 tbsps Lemon Juice
- 1 tbsp Maple Syrup
- 1 1/2 tsps Lemon Zest
- 1 tsp Vanilla Extract
- 1/16 tsp Sea Salt (optional)

INSTRUCTIONS

1. Add the shredded coconut to a food processor and blend until a coarse crumb forms.

2. Add the remaining ingredients to the shredded coconut in the food processor and blend until a dough forms. Form into even balls with your hands, roughly 1-inch in diameter.

3. Let them set in the fridge for at least an hour before serving. Store in the fridge or freezer until ready to enjoy.

NUTRITION - AMOUNT PER SERVING

Calories	152	Sugar	4g
Fat	14g	Protein	1g
Carbs	9g	Cholesterol	0mg
Fiber	3g	Sodium	37mg

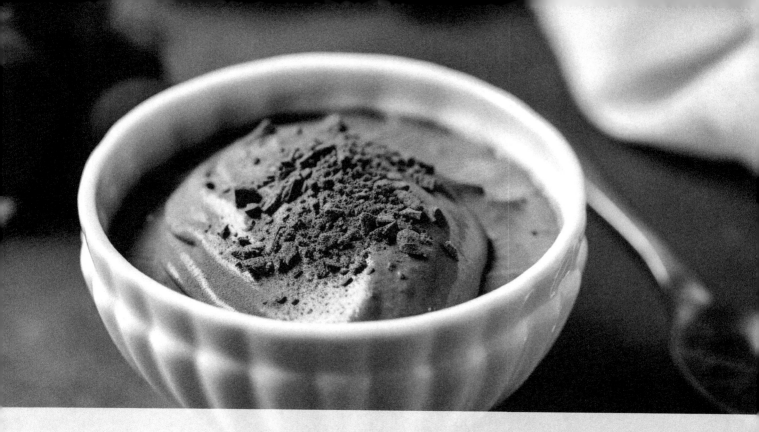

Dark Chocolate Peanut Mousse

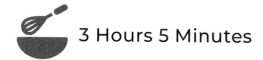 3 Hours 5 Minutes

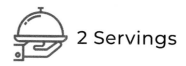 2 Servings

INGREDIENTS

- 2 cups Unsweetened Almond Milk
- 2 tbsps Chia Seeds
- 2 tsps Cocoa Powder
- ¼ cup All Natural Peanut Butter
- 3 tbsps Maple Syrup
- 1 tsp Vanilla Extract
- ½ tsp Sea Salt

INSTRUCTIONS

1. Place all the ingredients in a blender and blend for 2 to 3 minutes until a thickened, smooth, and creamy texture is achieved.

2. Transfer the mixture to a bowl once blended, and refrigerate until it is chilled, typically about three hours.

NUTRITION - AMOUNT PER SERVING

Calories	366	Sugar	22g
Fat	23g	Protein	11g
Carbs	35g	Cholesterol	0mg
Fiber	7g	Sodium	762mg

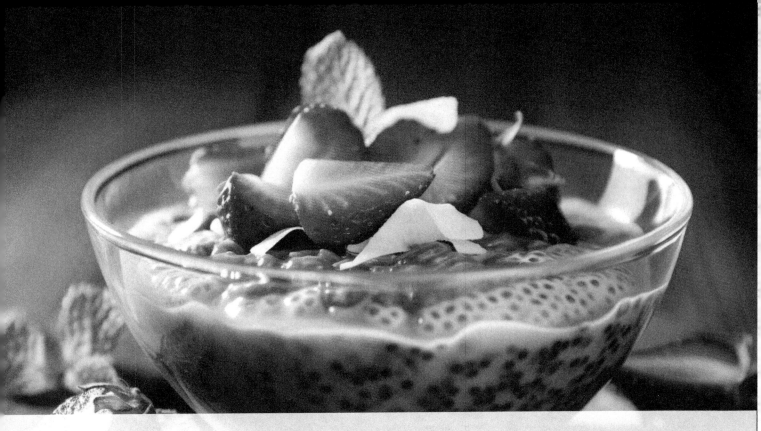

Coconut Yoghurt Chia Pudding

 30 Minutes

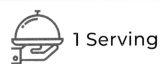 1 Serving

INGREDIENTS

- ½ cup Unsweetened Coconut Yogurt
- 2 tbsps Chia Seeds
- ¼ cup Unsweetened Almond Milk
- ½ cup Frozen Strawberries
- 1 tbsp All Natural Peanut Butter

INSTRUCTIONS

1. In a medium-sized bowl, add the yogurt, chia seeds, almond milk, and strawberries and stir well to combine.

2. Place in the fridge for 25 to 30 minutes, until thickened.

3. Remove from the fridge and stir in the peanut butter. Serve and enjoy!

NUTRITION - AMOUNT PER SERVING

Calories	1310	Sugar	7g
Fat	20g	Protein	9g
Carbs	30g	Cholesterol	0mg
Fiber	13g	Sodium	73mg

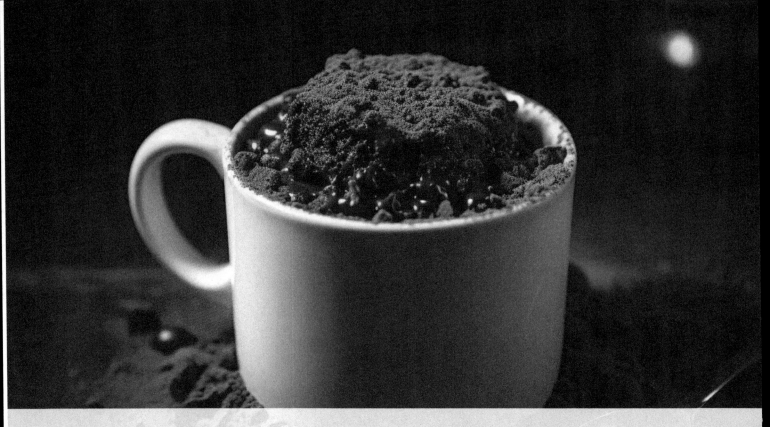

Double Chocolate Mug Cake

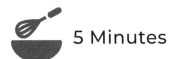 5 Minutes

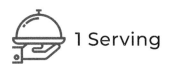 1 Serving

INGREDIENTS

- 2 tbsps Brown Rice Flour
- 2 tsps Cocoa Powder
- ¼ tsp Baking Powder
- 20 grams Dark Chocolate Chips
- 3 tbsps Unsweetened Almond Milk
- 1 ½ tbsps Maple Syrup
- 1 tbsp Avocado Oil

INSTRUCTIONS

1. In a mug combine the flour, cocoa powder, baking powder, and chocolate chips. Add the unsweetened almond milk, maple syrup, and oil. Stir well to combine.

2. Microwave for 90 seconds until the cake is spongy to the touch. Allow the mug cake to cool slightly and enjoy!

NUTRITION - AMOUNT PER SERVING

Calories	408	Sugar	28g
Fat	22g	Protein	4g
Carbs	48g	Cholesterol	0mg
Fiber	2g	Sodium	158mg

Smoothies

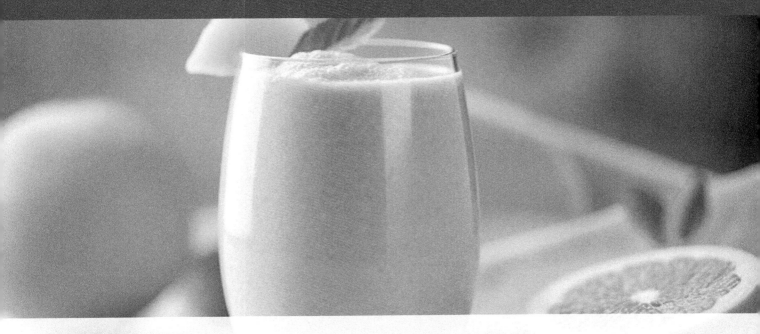

Orange Cantaloupe Smoothie

 5 Minutes

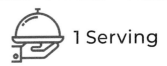 1 Serving

INGREDIENTS

- 1/4 Cantaloupe (small, chopped)
- 1/2 Navel Orange (peeled)
- 1/2 cup Water
- 1/2 cup Canned Coconut Milk
- 2 tbsps Unsweetened Coconut Yogurt
- 5 Ice Cubes

INSTRUCTIONS

1. Add all of the ingredients into a blender and blend until smooth.
2. Pour into a glass and enjoy!

NUTRITION - AMOUNT PER SERVING

Calories	307	Sugar	18g
Fat	22g	Protein	3g
Carbs	25g	Cholesterol	0mg
Fiber	3g	Sodium	62mg

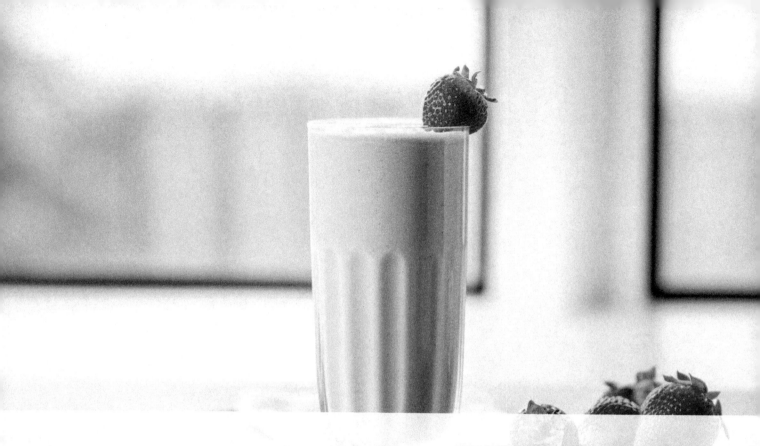

Strawberry & Peanut Butter Smoothie

 5 Minutes

 1 Serving

INGREDIENTS

- ¾ cup Unsweetened Almond Milk
- ½ cup Unsweetened Coconut Yogurt
- 65 grams Frozen Strawberries
- 1 tbsp All Natural Peanut Butter

INSTRUCTIONS

1. Add all ingredients to a blender and blend until smooth.
2. Pour into a glass and enjoy!

NUTRITION - AMOUNT PER SERVING

Calories	195	Sugar	5g
Fat	14g	Protein	5g
Carbs	16g	Cholesterol	0mg
Fiber	4g	Sodium	149mg

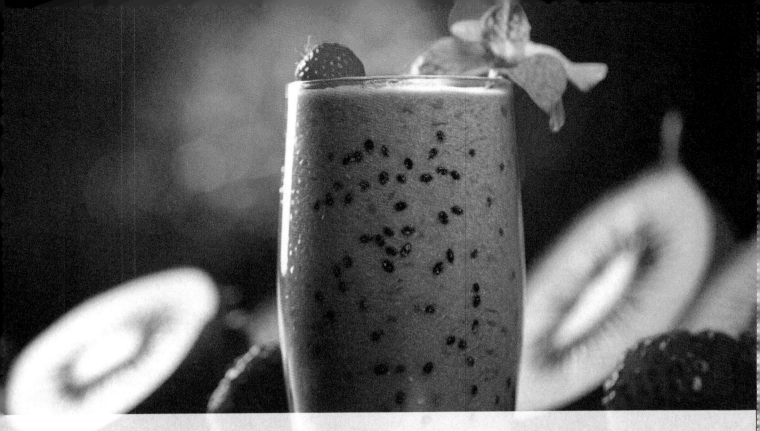

Dragon Fruit & Kiwi Smoothie

 5 Minutes

 1 Serving

INGREDIENTS

- 1/2 cup Plain Coconut Milk (unsweetened from the carton)
- 113 grams Dragon Fruit (red, cubed, fresh or frozen)
- 1/2 Kiwi
- 1/2 Lime (juiced)
- 1 tsp Maple Syrup
- 5 Ice Cubes

INSTRUCTIONS

1. Add all of the ingredients into a blender and blend until smooth.
2. Pour into a glass and enjoy!

NUTRITION - AMOUNT PER SERVING

Calories	151	Sugar	20g
Fat	3g	Protein	2g
Carbs	30g	Cholesterol	0mg
Fiber	4g	Sodium	20mg

Snacks

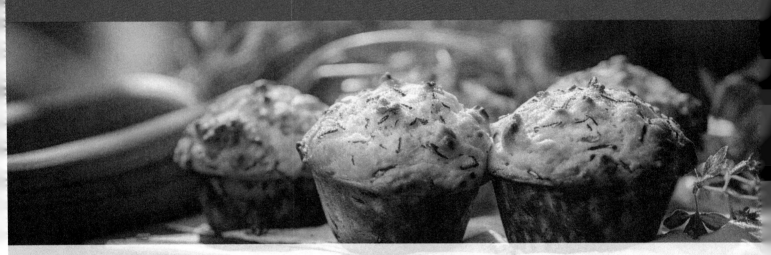

Zucchini Parmesan Muffins

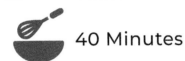 40 Minutes

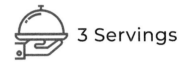 3 Servings

INGREDIENTS

- 75 grams Zucchini (sliced)
- Sea Salt & Black Pepper (to taste)
- ¼ cup Parmigiano Reggiano (finely grated)
- 2 Eggs
- ¼ cup Unsweetened Almond Milk
- 1 tbsp Butter (melted)
- ¼ cup Brown Rice Flour
- 1 tsp Baking Powder

INSTRUCTIONS

1. Preheat the oven to 350°F (175°C). Line a muffin tray with paper liners or use a silicone muffin tray.
2. Pat the zucchini slices dry with a paper towel. Transfer the zucchini to a bowl. Add salt, pepper, and parmesan cheese. Mix well.
3. In another bowl, add the milk, eggs, and butter. Whisk until everything is combined.
4. Sift the flour and baking powder together in a separate bowl. Then, whisk in the wet ingredients and combine well before folding in the zucchinis.
5. Evenly divide the batter between the muffin cups, approximately ⅓ cup per muffin. Transfer to the tray to the oven. Bake for 35 minutes until the muffins are cooked and golden brown.
6. Serve warm and enjoy!

NUTRITION - AMOUNT PER SERVING

Calories	174	Sugar	1g
Fat	10g	Protein	9g
Carbs	12g	Cholesterol	142mg
Fiber	1g	Sodium	286mg

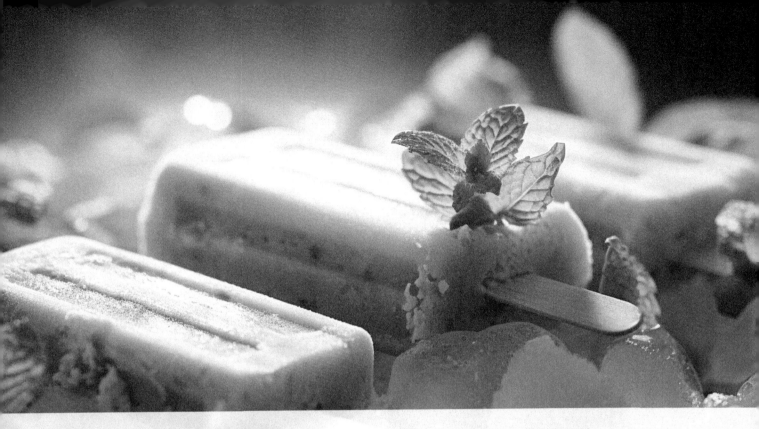

Vanilla Mint Matcha Creamsicles

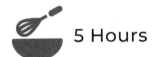 5 Hours

 2 Servings

INGREDIENTS

- 1/4 cup Canned Coconut Milk (full fat)
- 120 grams Unsweetened Coconut Yogurt
- 2 tbsps Maple Syrup
- 1 tbsp Vanilla Extract
- 1/3 cup Mint Leaves
- 2 tsps Green Tea Powder

INSTRUCTIONS

1. Combine all ingredients in a blender and blend for a minute or until smooth and creamy.

2. Pour into popsicle molds and transfer to the freezer to set for at least five hours.

NUTRITION - AMOUNT PER SERVING

Calories	156	Sugar	14g
Fat	7g	Protein	1g
Carbs	19g	Cholesterol	0mg
Fiber	1g	Sodium	25mg

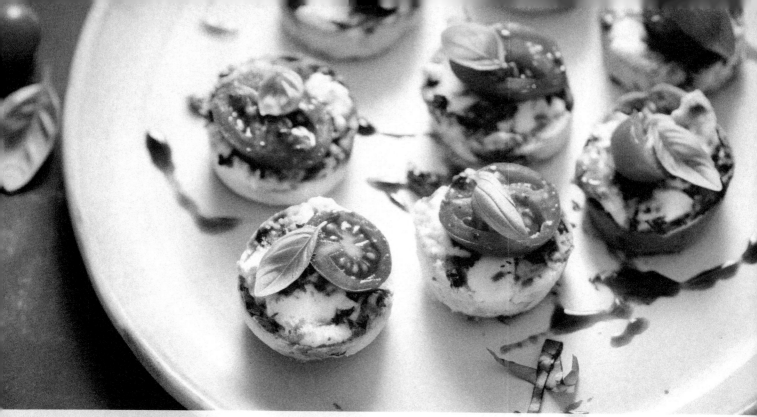

Balsamic Tomato & Basil Mini Egg White Bites

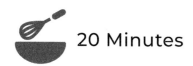 20 Minutes

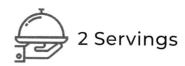 2 Servings

INGREDIENTS

- ½ cup Egg Whites
- 1 Tomato (medium, diced, juices drained)
- ½ cup Basil Leaves (chopped)
- 1 ½ tsps Balsamic Vinegar
- ⅛ tsp Sea Salt

INSTRUCTIONS

1. Preheat the oven to 350°F (175°C).
2. In a bowl, combine the egg whites, tomato, basil, balsamic vinegar, and salt.
3. Scoop the mixture into lined (or greased) mini muffin cups. Bake for 20 minutes or until cooked through. Let cool before serving.

NUTRITION - AMOUNT PER SERVING

Calories	46	Sugar	1g
Fat	0g	Protein	8g
Carbs	3g	Cholesterol	0mg
Fiber	1g	Sodium	273mg

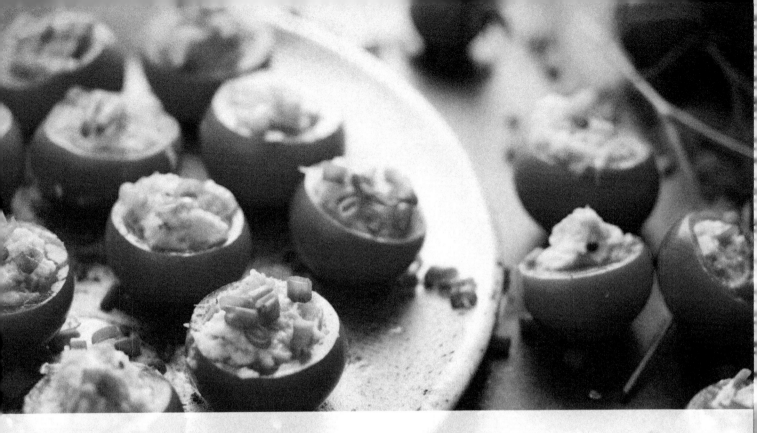

Salmon Stuffed Cherry Tomatoes

 25 Minutes

 3 Servings

INGREDIENTS

- 2 cups Cherry Tomatoes
- 106 grams Canned Wild Salmon
- 1 tbsp Dijon Mustard
- Sea Salt & Black Pepper (to taste)

INSTRUCTIONS

1. Cut the tops off of the cherry tomatoes and scoop out the insides. Discard or save for another dish.

2. Add the salmon, mustard, salt and pepper to a bowl and mix until well combined.

3. Stuff each tomato with the salmon mixture until it is all used up.

NUTRITION - AMOUNT PER SERVING

Calories	179	Sugar	3g
Fat	2g	Protein	10g
Carbs	4g	Cholesterol	23mg
Fiber	1g	Sodium	196mg

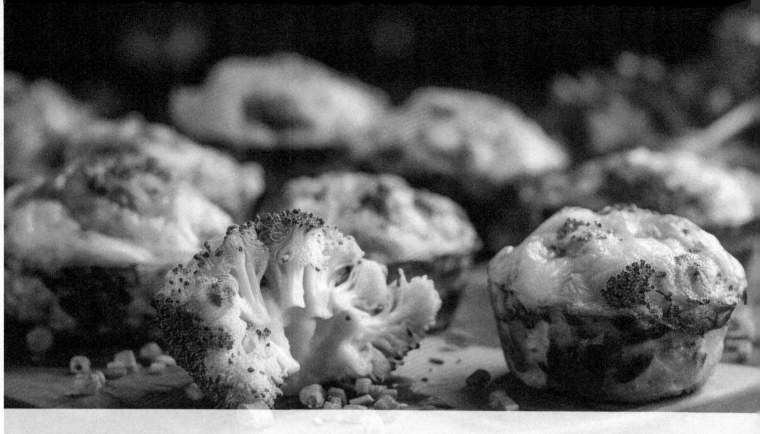

Broccoli & Cheddar Egg Muffins

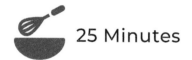 25 Minutes

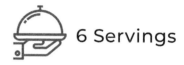 6 Servings

INGREDIENTS

- ½ cup Broccoli Florets (chopped)
- ½ Carrot (grated)
- 40 grams Cheddar Cheese (shredded)
- 5 Eggs (whisked)
- ¼ tsp Sea Salt

INSTRUCTIONS

1. Preheat the oven to 350°F (175°C). Grease a muffin tray or use a silicone muffin tray.

2. Evenly divide the broccoli, carrot, and cheese between the muffin cups of the prepared muffin tray.

3. Mix the eggs and salt together before pouring into the muffin tray. Bake for about 18 to 20 minutes until the eggs are cooked through. Let cool for 5 minutes.

NUTRITION - AMOUNT PER SERVING

Calories	91	Sugar	1g
Fat	6g	Protein	7g
Carbs	2g	Cholesterol	162mg
Fiber	0g	Sodium	207mg

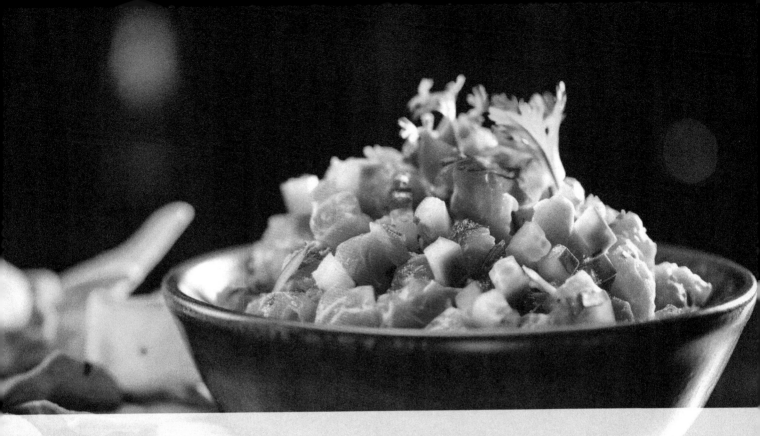

Salmon Tartare & Tortilla Chips

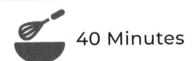 40 Minutes

 1 Serving

INGREDIENTS

- 113 grams Salmon Fillet (sushi-grade, skinless)
- 1/4 Cucumber (finely chopped)
- 1/4 Jalapeno Pepper (finely chopped)
- 1 tsp Avocado Oil
- 1/4 Lime (juiced and zested)
- 1 tsp Cilantro (finely chopped)
- Sea Salt & Black Pepper (to taste)
- 1 cup Corn Tortilla Chips

INSTRUCTIONS

1. Wrap the salmon in plastic wrap and place in the freezer for 30 minutes to firm up.

2. Remove the salmon from the plastic wrap and finely chop it into small cubes and then transfer to a bowl.

3. Add the cucumber, jalapeño, oil, lime juice, lime zest, and cilantro to the salmon and toss to combine. Season with salt and pepper. Serve with chips.

NUTRITION - AMOUNT PER SERVING

Calories	334	Sugar	2g
Fat	16g	Protein	28g
Carbs	21g	Cholesterol	58mg
Fiber	2g	Sodium	94mg

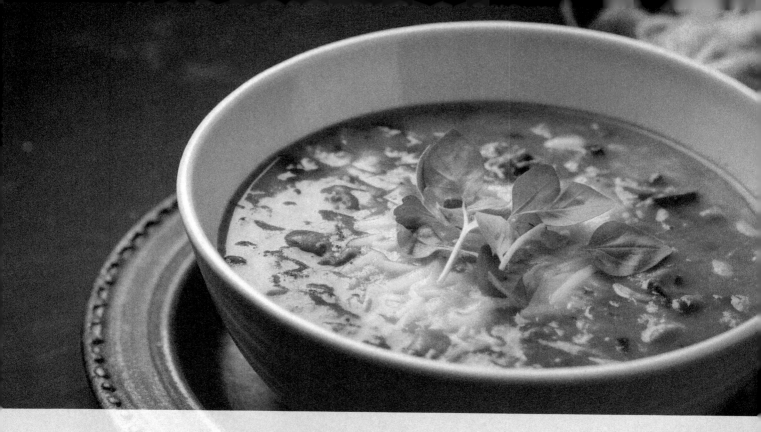

Cheeseburger Soup

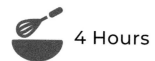 4 Hours

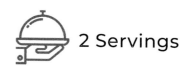 2 Servings

INGREDIENTS

- ¾ cup Beef Broth
- ⅓ cup Unsweetened Almond Milk
- ¼ tsp Dried Basil
- ⅛ Zucchini (chopped)
- Sea Salt & Black Pepper (to taste)
- 136 grams Extra Lean Ground Beef
- 45 grams Cheddar Cheese (shredded)

INSTRUCTIONS

1. Switch on the slow cooker and add the beef broth, almond milk, basil, zucchini, salt, and pepper.

2. Heat a nonstick pan over medium-high heat. Cook the ground beef for 5 to 8 minutes, breaking it up as it cooks. Drain extra fat if needed. Add the ground beef to the slow cooker and cook on low for four hours.

3. Divide the soup into bowls and top with cheddar cheese.

NUTRITION - AMOUNT PER SERVING

Calories	223	Sugar	1g
Fat	15g	Protein	20g
Carbs	2g	Cholesterol	66mg
Fiber	0g	Sodium	414mg

Food Translations

Depending on where you are in the world, some foods are known by different names. If you see an ingredient that you are not familiar with, check the chart below to see if it has a name you will recognize.

USA	UK	AUSTRALIA
ALL PURPOSE FLOUR	PLAIN FLOUR	PLAIN FLOUR
ARUGULA	ROCKET	ROCKET
BEETS	BEETROOT	BEETROOT
BELL PEPPERS	PEPPERS	CAPSICUM
CANTALOUPE	MELON	ROCK MELON
CILANTRO	CORIANDER	CORIANDER / CILANTRO
COLLARD GREENS	GREENS	GREENS
CORNSTARCH	CORNFLOUR	CORNFLOUR
EGGPLANT	AUBERGINE	EGGPLANT
SNOW PEAS	MANGETOUT	SNOW PEAS
GARBANZO BEANS	CHICKPEAS	CHICKPEAS
GROUND BEEF	MINCED BEEF	MINCE
PAPAYA	PAW PAW	PAW PAW
PINTO BEANS	SPECKLED BEANS	SPECKLED BEANS
POWDERED SUGAR	ICING SUGAR	ICING SUGAR
ROMAINE LETTUCE	COS LETTUCE	COS LETTUCE
RUTABAGA	SWEDE	SWEDE
SCALLIONS	SPRING ONIONS	SPRING ONIONS
SHRIMP	PRAWN	PRAWN
SWISS CHARD	CHARD	SILVERBEET
ZUCCHINI	COURGETTE	ZUCCHINI

Cooking Conversions

CUP	ONCES	MILLILITERS	TBSP
8 cup	64 oz	1895 ml	128
6 cup	48 oz	1420 ml	96
5 cup	40 oz	1180 ml	80
4 cup	32 oz	960 ml	64
2 cup	16 oz	500 ml	32
1 cup	8 oz	250 ml	16
3/4 cup	6 oz	177 ml	12
2/3 cup	5 oz	158 ml	11
1/2 cup	4 oz	118 ml	8
3/8 cup	3 oz	90 ml	6
1/3 cup	2.5 oz	79 ml	5.5
1/4 cup	2 oz	59 ml	4
1/8 cup	1 oz	30 ml	3
1/16 cup	1/2 oz	15 ml	1

IMPERIAL	METRIC
1/2 oz	15 g
1 oz	29 g
2 oz	57 g
3 oz	85 g
4 oz	113 g
5 oz	141 g
6 oz	170 g
8 oz	227 g
10 oz	283 g
12 oz	340 g
13 oz	369 g
14 oz	397 g
15 oz	425 g
1 lb	453 g

FAHRENHEIT	CELSIUS
100 °F	37 °C
150 °F	65 °C
200 °F	93 °C
250 °F	121 °C
300 °F	150 °C
325 °F	160 °C
350 °F	180 °C

FAHRENHEIT	CELSIUS
350 °F	180 °C
375 °F	190 °C
400 °F	200 °C
425 °F	220 °C
450 °F	230 °C
500 °F	260 °C
525 °F	274 °C
550 °F	288 °C

Printed in Great Britain
by Amazon

37242417R00123